Designing and Teaching Online Courses in Nursing

Sally Kennedy, PhD, APRN, FNP, CNE, is a semi-retired lifelong learner who is committed to reforming online education. She recently retired as an assistant professor to pursue consulting and writing. Dr. Kennedy has been a nurse for more than 40 years, with most of her career spent in clinical practice as a nurse practitioner. When she began teaching nurse practitioner students 20 years ago, she became enthralled with teaching methods and subsequently pursued a doctorate in online education with a specialization in online instructional design. Along the way, Dr. Kennedy was introduced to problem-based learning (PBL), realized its potential for clinical nursing education, and subsequently led faculty in the transition from a master's-level, classroom-based PBL curriculum to an online program, which *U.S. News & World Report* recognized as number one among online graduate nursing programs.

Designing and Teaching Online Courses in Nursing

Sally Kennedy, PhD, APRN, FNP, CNE

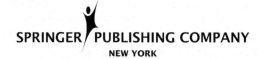

SPRINGER PUBLISHING COMPANY
NEW YORK

Springer Publishing Company, LLC
11 West 42nd Street
New York, NY 10036
www.springerpub.com

Acquisitions Editor: Joseph Morita
Compositor: Westchester Publishing Services

ISBN: 978-0-8261-3408-0
e-book ISBN: 978-0-8261-3409-7
Supplemental template ISBN: 978-0-8261-3374-8

Supplemental templates are available from www.springerpub.com/kennedy

17 18 19 20 21/ 5 4 3 2 1

The author and the publisher of this Work have made every effort to use sources believed to be reliable to provide information that is accurate and compatible with the standards generally accepted at the time of publication. Because medical science is continually advancing, our knowledge base continues to expand. Therefore, as new information becomes available, changes in procedures become necessary. We recommend that the reader always consult current research and specific institutional policies before performing any clinical procedure. The author and publisher shall not be liable for any special, consequential, or exemplary damages resulting, in whole or in part, from the readers' use of, or reliance on, the information contained in this book. The publisher has no responsibility for the persistence or accuracy of URLs for external or third-party Internet websites referred to in this publication and does not guarantee that any content on such websites is, or will remain, accurate or appropriate.

Library of Congress Cataloging-in-Publication Data
Names: Kennedy, Sally, author.
Title: Designing and teaching online courses in nursing / Sally Kennedy.
Description: New York, NY: Springer Publishing Company, LLC, [2017] |
    Includes bibliographical references and index.
Identifiers: LCCN 2017002561 | ISBN 9780826134080 (hardcopy: alk. paper) |
    ISBN 9780826134097 (ebook)
Subjects: | MESH: Education, Nursing—methods | Education, Distance—methods
Classification: LCC RT71 | NLM WY 18 | DDC 610.73071/1—dc23 LC record available at
    https://lccn.loc.gov/2017002561

Printed in the United States of America by Gasch Printing.

For my husband,
Milt Dodge

Contents

Preface

It is hard to believe that the call to reform nursing education came more than 5 years ago with the publication of *Educating Nurses: A Call for Radical Transformation* (Benner, Sutphen, Leonard, & Day, 1984/2010). However, as is true to my experience in the profession and the past 50 years of nursing history, we are not a group of early adopters. Yet, today, online education is upon us as evidenced by the rise in popularity of online RN to bachelor of science in nursing (BSN), master's, doctor of nursing practice (DNP), and PhD programs. Driven by economic issues, the nursing shortage, adult learners with responsibilities beyond their careers, and technology, more and more nursing educators—like it or not—are faced with teaching online.

As with teaching in the classroom, the assumption has been that teaching online will just come naturally. After all, most of our current nursing educators learned to teach by the apprenticeship method; they learned from a seasoned educator. This has worked for decades, but the philosophy of teaching and the educational theories that support it have changed—or, more accurately, we are now becoming aware of and working to implement these changes. Although lecturing has been the teaching method used for decades, we can no longer ignore constructivism, social constructivism, and findings from cognitive psychology research that have recently been translated and made understandable for the average educator (Brown, Roediger, & McDaniel, 2014; Miller, 2014).

Online education has made it possible not only to operationalize a constructivist learning environment, but also to create learning opportunities that recognize and build upon the knowledge and skills the adult learner brings to it. However, most nursing educators must rely on their commitment to lifelong learning to become proficient with strategies available for teaching online. If they are fortunate, they can learn from a seasoned online educator. The apprenticeship method remains alive and well.

In this how-to book, I have outlined the steps I see as necessary to accomplish the call to transform nursing education, specifically, contextualizing knowledge and understandings (knowing *that*) with knowing *how, when,* and *why* to mimic the complexities of nursing practice, be that from a clinical, research, administrative, or educational perspective. As a result of their education, students must be able to employ multiple ways of thinking consistent with their new role, extract salient information in changing and unstable situations, and develop an evidence-based plan and see it through. We must not only teach the knowledge, skills, and attitudes necessary to accomplish this, but also help students gain the ability to use these tools in flexible ways.

This transformation will require more than simply replacing the lecture with online discussions. It will involve rethinking how we teach, moving away from a content-focused, teacher-driven perspective to one that is outcome focused and learning driven. The process must begin by changing how objectives are written and how we view teaching and assessing. Not-so-recent research from cognitive psychology can guide us, and you might be surprised how.

In writing this book I have drawn from my experience working as an instructional designer teaching faculty how to teach online. Most of these educators had little theoretical background in educational theories, models, and concepts and lacked a solid understanding of how to operationalize these online. Research from cognitive psychology has been difficult to interpret, and then translate into effective teaching strategies, until recently with the understandable synthesis of research published by Brown, Roediger, and McDaniel (2014) and the practical application to teaching for higher education found in the work of Miller (2014).

In Chapters 1 and 2 of this book, my goal was to start with an even playing field by discussing what I consider foundational theories and concepts related to who our learners are and how they learn, introducing how research from cognitive science can help us create opportunities for deep, long-term learning. The testing effect, spaced study, and "interleaving" may be new concepts for many, but what they can teach us about how people learn will amaze you.

When planning an online course, backward is best. By that I mean using the process of Backward Design (Wiggins & McTighe, 2005) to design your online course, *starting* with outcomes instead of *covering* content. This approach maintains your focus on learning, not teaching, and puts assessment in a prominent place that shares its position with teaching methods, as the two cannot be separated when teaching online. More on that appears in Chapter 3, where you will also find some very practical information on the elements of online course design and how workload impacts that.

Although writing behavioral objectives for your course may seem like old news, we must approach them differently if we are to transform nursing education. As Chapter 4 reminds us, objectives drive what is taught and learned, so only by communicating the desired learning outcome of integrated performance will that be realized.

Teaching and assessment are one activity when teaching online; they are not separate activities and cannot be considered as two unrelated processes. This is an important concept to grasp, especially if you are a seasoned classroom instructor accustomed to creating separate assessments that add to your workload. Chapter 5 explores how this interconnected approach works. Online small group discussions serve as both formative and summative assessment; these discussions are engaging for students as they wrestle with complex questions and real-life case studies that have them thinking like a nurse practitioner, administrator, researcher, or educator—whichever role they aspire to. Creating engaging discussion questions and case studies is your job, which is so vital to teaching online that I devoted two chapters to these topics (see Chapters 6 and 7). Chapter 8 details methods for effective online testing using multiple-choice questions, which take advantage of the testing effect, creating additional opportunities for teaching and learning.

Grading is an important function that drives learning and deserves some attention, as I think we have lost our way to some degree when assessing what constitutes academic achievement. Rubrics have replaced other grading strategies, but not all meet the expectation of greater objectivity in grading, which is their initial intent. Chapter 9 is presented to reorient educators to the value and intent of this grading tool by reiterating the three components that define a rubric. Included in this chapter are step-by-step instructions on how to create a rubric in Excel, add formulas to compute a grade, and save grading time.

A hot topic in online education that relates to workload is the expectation of faculty presence in an online course from both faculty's and the student's perspective. This topic is explored in Chapter 10. What is currently recommended may shock you, but if my recommendations throughout the book are followed when designing your online course, daily presence is not so daunting. To help you be present in your course, meet students' expectations, yet not become the center of the discussion, facilitation strategies, as described in Chapter 11, provide some useful tools.

For many faculty, technology adds an often unwanted challenge when starting to teach online. Learning management systems (LMSs) that house online courses have similar functionality, so if you learn one, learning the next is not as difficult. In Chapter 12, I provide tips on interface design that will help you create a user-friendly course with consistent navigation so students can focus on learning and not spend hours trying to find information.

Converting a classroom-based course to the online environment can be a time-consuming task when you do not have some guidance as to where to start. Online education is more than uploading your classroom lectures into the LMS. Lengthy lectures, particularly those that reiterate the assigned readings, simply have no place online. However, they can be useful in planning learning activities and assessments. In Chapter 13, I provide a step-wise approach with some additional tips on converting a classroom course to the online environment, based on many concepts discussed in earlier chapters in the book.

This book differs from most others related to teaching online because it takes a how-to approach with the dual goals of answering the call to transform nursing education and benefiting from research in cognitive psychology. Each chapter includes relevant concepts, theories, and models to guide course design and teaching online, as well as practical tips and pearls. Included in the Appendix are templates that provide a means of organizing your thoughts as you design your online course or convert a classroom course to the online environment. Reviewing these templates in the Appendix will give you a better idea of what I am referring to in the text of the various chapters. **So that you do not have to re-create the wheel, these templates are also available for download in Word format (.docx) from the Springer Publishing Company website at www.springerpub .com/kennedy. They can be used "as is" or customized to meet your needs. Also available online is an example of a rubric in Excel, and a one-page tutorial on how to use this.**

In addition, this book is written informally, moving away from the impersonal third person typically found in nursing texts. I wanted this to be more of a conversation with the readers, indicating that we are in this together. I have attempted to learn from cognitive psychology, taking advantage of spaced education and the interleaving technique that you will read about in Chapter 2 by repeating important concepts and adding to them in the process. So, you will notice some repetition, which was done by design.

Sally Kennedy

REFERENCES

Benner, P., Sutphen, M., Leonard, V., & Day, L. (1984/2010). *Educating nurses: A call for radical transformation* [Commemorative ed.]. San Francisco, CA: Jossey-Bass.

Brown, P. C., Roediger, H. L., III, & McDaniel, M. A. (2014). *Make it stick: The science of successful learning*. Cambridge, MA: Belknap Press.

Miller, M. D. (2014). *Minds online: Teaching effectively with technology*. Cambridge, MA: Harvard University Press.

Wiggins, G., & McTighe, J. (2005). *Understanding by design* (2nd ed.). Alexandria, VA: Association for Supervision and Curriculum Development.

Acknowledgments

Writing a book, I discovered, takes time, perseverance, and the support of many. Were it not for the continued encouragement from my husband, Milt Dodge, who understood the joy I felt while researching and writing even though it meant countless hours on his own, this book would not have been written. He endured many hours of listening to educational theory and its application as I endeavored to find the words to explain (to myself) what seemed so intuitive to me, but which my experience working with faculty taught me often was not. Although his eyes sometimes glazed over, he listened intently and provided feedback when possible, but most of all he believed in my ability to pull it together when I had temporarily lost faith in my ability to do so. I am so blessed to have him by my side.

I am indebted to the entire publishing staff at Springer Publishing Company, including Joseph Morita, senior acquisitions editor, who saw value in my proposal; Rachel Landes, assistant editor, who was an invaluable resource for a first-time book author; Donna Frassetto, content development specialist, for her helpful comments and encouragement; and Lindsay Claire, managing editor, who expertly guided a novice throughout the production process. They have all been amazing to work with!

I would also like to thank Pamela Lankas for her proofreading expertise and Sivakumar Kathiresan, project manager at Antares Publishing Services, a subsidiary of Westchester Publishing Services, for his attention to detail in transforming a manuscript into a book. That was so exciting to see!

Professionally, I would like to thank Dr. Anna Cianciolo, associate professor, Department of Medical Education, Southern Illinois School of Medicine, for pointing me in a fruitful direction with regard to published articles on problem-based learning. In addition, the librarians at the Charles Trumbull Hayden Library and Noble Science and Engineering Library at Arizona State University, my alma mater, remained cheerful when answering my many questions. Their expert advice and direction saved countless hours of wandering through the stacks and searching online. A heartfelt thank you to all!

And, I must include a heartfelt tribute to my furry companion, Brewster, who stayed by my side and kept me company throughout the many hours, days, and months I worked on this book. I know he is happy and romping with his cousin, Harley, by the rainbow bridge where we will meet again one day.

1

Our Learners and How They Learn

GENERATIONS ONLINE

For the first time in history, students from three generations could conceivably be found taking classes in college. These generations are the baby boomers, Gen-Xers, and millennials. Much has been written about the Gen-Xers and millennials with regard to personality traits, expectations of life, how they learn, and other dimensions on how they differ from previous college students. I have been tempted to reiterate the information. However, other, more relevant forces are at work in higher education, such as moving education from the classroom to the online environment, a change that many faculty are ill-prepared for from a theoretical and practical perspective; recent findings about how the brain works with relation to learning; the use of handheld technology as peripheral cognitive storage; and the not-so-recent understandings from the field of cognitive psychology that are being translated into practice in higher education. Thus, I will resist the urge to summarize what has been written about these groups as the information seems to be a moving target. Instead, let me place these generations in perspective chronologically.

Before providing a brief overview of the three generations, sans characteristics, understanding what the terms *traditional* and *nontraditional* learners mean is in order. Not specifically defined, but almost universally understood without using the term "traditional," these students enrolled full time in college immediately after graduation from high school and were financially dependent upon others, typically their parents. Conversely, the concept of the nontraditional student has been the focus of research on persistence and risk of attrition, although a consensus for a definition of the "nontraditional" student has not been reached (Chung, Turnbull, & Chur-Hansen, 2014). Studies completed for the National Center for Education Statistics (NCES; Radford, Cominole, & Skomsvold, 2015) used the following characteristics to identify undergraduate nontraditional learners:

- Delaying college enrollment until age 24
- Part-time enrollment
- Working full time while attending school
- Financially independent (i.e., not reliant on support from their parents)
- Responsible for at least one dependent
- Being a single parent
- Earning a general equivalency diploma instead of a high school diploma

Findings from five separate NCES studies from 1995 to 2012 on the nontraditional learner have been consistent over time and indicate that 74% of college students can be defined as nontraditional.

The distinction between traditional and nontraditional students may have greater implications for teaching and learning than generational differences. Most online nursing programs involve either RN to bachelor of science in nursing (BSN) or graduate students. These students will, most likely, fit the definition of the nontraditional learner because they work more than 35 hours each week and are financially independent. They may also be single parents. This characterization has implications for the time they can devote to studying, which encourages faculty to choose teaching strategies and assessments strategically, as well as to design the learning management system (LMS) for intuitive navigation.

Baby Boomers

The baby boomers were born between 1945 and 1964, which means the *youngest* members of this group turned 50 in 2014. Some of these students may very well return to college for a second career or graduate study. Most likely, they are traditional learners who were taught in the classroom, where lecture was the main educational strategy used.

Many nursing faculty belong to this generation. Recent national statistics indicate that the average age of doctorally prepared nursing faculty, regardless of rank, and the average age of full professors at 61.6 years old (American Association of Colleges of Nursing [AACN], 2014). In addition, 50% of RNs—and therefore potential students—are older than 50 years of age, according to a survey by the National Council of the State Boards of Nursing (2013).

Gen-X

Gen-Xers, the children of the baby boomers, were so named because some authors felt, as a group, they lacked a generation-defining event (Wilson, 2002). Sandwiched in-between the boomers and millennials, they are considered traditional learners even though they grew up with technology. Although authors differ on exact dates, the Gen-Xers were born from the mid-1960s to the early 1980s. The *oldest* members of this group turned 50 in 2015.

Millennials

The millennials were born between the early 1980s and 2004, although some authors are less solid on the dates. Technology has been with this group their entire lives, with many using computers from a very early age. The oldest members of this group are in their early 30s, the youngest in middle school.

A plethora of writing has been published on the Net Generation (Gen-Xers and millennials), much of it in disagreement, leaving the educator with few solid strategies to advise teaching. Instead of attempting to customize our teaching to meet disparate characteristics of our learners, our focus should be on applying effective learning theories, models, and concepts, regardless of how long they have been around; using teaching strategies that support how the mind learns, regardless of how old or what generation that mind belongs to; and using technology effectively and efficiently to support all of this. Thus, the focus of this chapter is on the learners and how they learn, introducing concepts that have been around for a while, but perhaps may be less familiar to nurse educators. In addition, I discuss perhaps even less familiar concepts to promote learning from cognitive science research.

The Net Generation

Another means of identifying traditional and nontraditional learners is how they learn, which for the Gen-Xers and millennials is technology based, leading many to prefer the more descriptive term of *Net Generation* for these two generational groups. Although not true for all members of the Net Generation, they have come to rely on technology in all aspects of their lives, including learning, which led Rosen (2011) to define a subgroup of the Net Generation born in the 1990s that he calls the *iGeneration*. For this group, technology is not something special to be used under specific circumstances. Instead, all forms of technology—laptops, tablets, smartphones, e-readers, and so forth—are extensions of who they are; a very different perspective from how the telephone was thought of by the baby boomers. In Rosen's (2011) view, members of the iGeneration "don't question the existence of technology and media. They expect technology to be there, and they expect it to do whatever they want it to do. Their WWW doesn't stand for World Wide Web; it stands for Whatever, Whenever, Wherever" (para. 7).

This perspective has the potential to forever alter how we teach and the definition of *learning* in general. Having the answer to almost any question a few clicks away by using a handheld device of some sort, learners have essentially added *external brain capacity*. This may alleviate the need to teach many facts and concepts, instead shifting the focus of education to critical thinking, critical appraisal, and the ability to distinguish reliable resources from those that are not. With this somewhat radical thought in mind, a review of what is currently known about how we learn is in order.

HOW WE LEARN

Learning occurs because of the interaction among attention, thinking, and memory. One cannot learn for the long term without attending to the lessons, engaging cognitive and metacognitive processes, and encoding and storing whatever was attended to in long-term memory (LTM). Our understanding of how learning occurs has shifted from what Miller (2014) refers to as the *three-box theory* of memory, specifically working memory, short-term memory (STM), and LTM, to that of the relationship of attention to memory.

The Three-Box Theory

Research on memory is in a bit of a flux, with the three-box theory falling out of favor and an explanation understandable to educators yet to emerge from cognitive research (Miller, 2014). The process originally introduced by Atkinson and Shiffrin (1968), which Miller (2014) refers to as the three-box theory, was composed of three subsystems, "sensory register, short-term store, and the long-term store" (p. 16), now known as working memory, STM, and LTM. Although gaps in our understanding exist, which explain how observations from our environment become mental representations that are then stored in memory, the current understanding is that "the brain converts your perceptions into chemical and electrical changes that form a mental representation of the patterns you've observed" (Brown, Roediger, & McDaniel, 2014, p. 72). How these mental representations became retrievable is illusive, but the process has been referred to as *encoding* since the early research of Tulving and Thomson (1973), and the representations are called *memory traces*. Through a process called *consolidation*, these memory traces are organized and linked to prior knowledge that helps make sense out of the incoming information. Consolidation may take hours to days to occur and is an unconscious phenomenon, resulting in storage in LTM as a *schema* or *mental model*. What strengthens the consolidation process is time away from actively thinking about the information, with sleep actually promoting the process.

Retrieval, recalling, or remembering the information is necessary to use the information. Retrieving information from LTM and moving it into working memory "can both strengthen the memory traces and at the same time make them modifiable again, enabling them, for example, to connect to more recent learning. This process is called reconsolidation. This is how retrieval practice modifies and strengthens learning" (Brown et al., 2014, p. 74). Cues, or aspects of the information (content and context), employed to store memories are important for retrieval. These cues are strengthened and new ones added through mental rehearsal, a means of recall or retrieval. Without periodic rehearsal or retrieval, over time the cues are forgotten. The memory remains, but it cannot be accessed and therefore is not retrieved without a cue to bring it forward. Remembering information within a context, however, provides a richer selection of cues that makes information easier to recall. Thus, learning requires encoding into LTM, making associations with multiple cues, and practicing retrieval so that the cues remain active (Brown et al., 2014).

Mental Models

Mental models can range from a single piece of data to a bundle of related knowledge *(know that)*, skills *(know how)*, and a complex set of connections that are difficult to extract, but have to do with applying the information, or *knowing when*. For example, as a child you might have a schema or mental model for a specific grocery store because your mother takes you to the same store shopping each week. As your experience increases, the concept of *grocery store* takes on a variety of meanings from a corner convenience store where a small selection of groceries can be purchased to a Walmart Supercenter that has just about everything. Yet, your mental model stored in LTM is that of a grocery store in general that contains multiple links or traces to various types of grocery stores. Mental models or schemas provide bundled storage in LTM, so as not to tax the capacity of working memory or STM. When the data is needed, we can retrieve it via the traces; bringing it back into consciousness for use. If we encounter a new piece of information, such as that grocery stores in Colorado do not sell alcohol, our mental model for grocery stores has just been modified.

Developing mental models takes practice and occurs over time, so it is not surprising that experts have more mental models than novices, which promote the fluid and intuitive performance of the expert. The news is not all good here, as experts often have difficulty deconstructing their mental models because the individual elements are so embedded in complex cognitive structures. Novices, after all, are rule-guided when applying what they have learned, which requires that they learn it in a step-wise fashion (Benner, 1984/2001; Brown et al., 2014).

Cognitive Load

The concept of cognitive load is built on the known limited capacity of working memory. Sweller, Van Merrienboer, and Paas (1998) explained that:

> because working memory is most commonly used to process information in the sense of organizing, contrasting, comparing, or working on that information in some manner, humans are probably only able to deal with two or three items of information simultaneously when required to process rather than merely hold information. (p. 252)

Here the authors make a distinction between holding information and actually processing it, which involves, among other activities, that of schema creation or modification. Three types of cognitive load have been identified as *intrinsic, extraneous,* and *germane* (Young, Van Merrienboer, Durning, & Ten Cate, 2014).

Intrinsic cognitive load is that imposed by course content itself. For example, if the course content is completely new to students, meaning they have no mental models or prior knowledge to fall back on, and contains multiple interrelated elements, then intrinsic load can be high. Faculty can do little to control for this other than assuring that assigned readings are consistent with the student's educational level, breaking complex content into smaller more understandable chunks, and choosing reading and assignments strategically.

Extraneous cognitive load is that imposed by the design and organization of learning materials and the online LMS (i.e., Moodle or Blackboard) that faculty *can* control. The extraneous cognitive load has to do with how the computer–user interface is designed and is discussed in Chapter 12. If the LMS is not well designed, students spend an inordinate amount of time trying to locate information. Also, if the syllabus and organization of the LMS are not parallel, additional extraneous cognitive load is imposed, a topic discussed in Chapter 12.

Two types of *extrinsic* cognitive load have been identified—*split attention* and *redundancy*—which have implications for choosing instructional resources for students. *Split attention* refers to providing multiple resources for the student to consider. If students' time is limited, which it often is for nontraditional students, choosing which resource to use, because they do not have time to read or review them all, adds extra cognitive load.

Consequently, students' attention is split among these resources, which may result in students feeling overwhelmed and not attending to any of them. *Redundancy* refers to providing repetitious resources. This is especially frustrating for students who prefer to make hard copies of references, resulting in wasted paper and printer ink.

Adaptive Memory Framework

Nairne, Thompson, and Pandeirada (2007) formulated a more recent theory of memory termed the *adaptive memory framework*, which posits that memory is evolutionary and adapts to remember what is most crucial to solving recurring problems related to survival and reproduction. The foundation of their theory is based on how the brain has adapted over time to ensure the survival of the species in a changing environment. Thus, its primary function has been that of remembering important information in order to solve problems.

How does this relate to teaching and learning? Nairne et al. (2007) views memory from a functional perspective as opposed to the structural view of the three-box theory. Their theory posits that we are most attuned to what we care about. This can be translated into our teaching practices by taking the time to determine what information students must know, what they believe is nice to know, and what is really irrelevant to their future goals. Miller (2014) suggests posing these questions to help you make a distinction among these three areas: "Why should students remember the information I'm giving them? Does it relate to their goals? . . . If not, they are likely to forget it—a case of the brain just doing its job the way evolution shaped it to do" (p. 98).

COGNITION, METACOGNITION, AND REFLECTION

Flavell (1979) first described the term *metacognition* as "cognition about cognitive phenomena" (p. 906). As *cognition* refers to thinking, metacognition is really *thinking about thinking*. Metacognition can be thought of as that internal voice that guides and monitors thinking and learning. I am sure you know what I mean—that little voice in your head that gets your attention to tell you it did not understand what you just read, for example.

Metacognition

Flavel (1979) identified three types of metacognition: knowledge about the self, knowledge about cognitive tasks, and strategic knowledge.

Self-knowledge requires knowing one's strengths and weaknesses to prepare for learning appropriately, being aware of the depth and breadth of one's knowledge, and understanding what strategies work best for specific learning tasks. Self-knowledge is related to motivation and self-efficacy, which also affect how students approach learning. It is this self-knowledge that leads to the concept of assessment driving learning, for students choose the appropriate study strategy depending on the perceived demands of how the material will be assessed, such as the type of test.

Knowledge about cognitive tasks encompasses the ability to recognize the complexity of a task. This includes matching that task with the appropriate learning strategy and understanding when and why particular strategies are appropriate.

Strategic knowledge is the most applicable in this context as it includes the specific strategies employed for learning and problem solving. Weinstein and Mayer (1983) have grouped these various strategies into five categories: *rehearsal, elaboration, organizational, comprehension monitoring,* and *affective.*

Rehearsal is an active, yet not particularly effective, form of learning in which the learner repeats information over and over in an attempt to memorize it. Rehearsal also involves highlighting content in the text or copying important information in notes. Highlighting information in a text to improve learning has been researched by cognitive scientists and found not to be particularly strategic for learning (Roediger, 2013).

Elaboration involves "paraphrasing, summarizing, or describing how new information relates to existing knowledge" (Weinstein & Mayer, 1983, para. 8) and serves to bring forth prior knowledge into working memory to assimilate it with the new information. Elaboration strategies are more effective than rehearsal strategies. Answering self-generated questions or completing those provided in the text is one of the elaboration strategies requiring retrieval from LTM that has been found to be effective for long-term learning and transfer (Brown et al., 2014).

Organizational strategies involve outlining a chapter, concept mapping, or diagraming. These activities serve to bring forth the relationships among and between elements of content (Weinstein & Mayer, 1983).

Comprehension-monitoring activities include those that check for understanding such as reviewing questions in a text *prior* to reading in order to focus the learner on important content and activate prior knowledge. This type of self-monitoring activity requires that the student set goals, monitor progress in meeting those goals, and modify strategies accordingly (Weinstein & Mayer, 1983).

Affective strategies involve monitoring anxiety levels or negative self-talk of failure to maintain focus on the task at hand and taking active steps to remain alert. Another affective strategy involves studying in a quiet place (Weinstein & Mayer, 1983).

Reflection

Nursing educators seem to focus on the term *reflection*, which is often equated with metacognition. Reflective journals and other reflective assignments are common in nursing and do serve as retrieval practice (Brown et al., 2014). The desired outcome of reflection is to improve practice based on a mental review of related knowledge and experience regarding a specific performance. A variety of models exist that include different language, but seem to agree that the purpose of reflection is to identify learning needs; integrate personal beliefs, attitudes, and values with knowledge and experience; and link what is known to new knowledge and experience (Mann, Gordon, & MacLeod, 2009).

Schön (1987), who first described the *reflective practitioner*, is also credited with separating the construct into reflection-*in*-action and reflection-*on*-action. *Reflection-in-action* is activated when the individual lacks adequate experience performing the task or the task is complex. This form of reflection may be considered parallel to metacognition for it involves *thinking about thinking during* the performance task to guide thoughts and actions. Reflection-in-action may result in modification of performance based on knowledge and prior experience combined with real-time environmental cues such as a patient's changing condition. This is difficult for the educator to assess while the performance is occurring, but afterward, the student can verbally walk faculty through what he or she was thinking while performing the task. Conducting research on this construct is equally challenging because what is occurring in the student's mind cannot be assessed as it is occurring (Mann et al., 2009).

Reflection-on-action is commonly used as an assignment in education as a means to encourage learning from experience. I do think that when the term *reflection* is used in this context it is this construct of reflection-on-action that is meant. Reflection in this regard occurs after the performance has been completed and requires critical thinking and analysis (Mann et al., 2009). This type of reflection includes revisiting the experience without constraints of time; experiencing the emotions felt during the event or when thinking about the event; and evaluating the experience in terms of how it fits with existing knowledge and experience. The outcome of reflection is to validate, reshape, and/or completely revise future performance (Boud, 2001).

Boud (2001) adds another dimension to reflection-in-action or reflection-on-action and that is *reflection-before-action*, or preparing oneself for what is to come. He specifies three aspects to this practice: focusing on the learner, the context, and potential learning to be gained. This pre-experience type of reflection brings into conscious awareness what the learner should consider and tune into to gain the most from the learning experience. This strategy is often employed during clinicals when a preceptor takes the student aside prior to performing a new skill to review the procedure, which results in both student and instructor feeling assured that the student is prepared for the task.

Taken together, the work of Schön and Boud was combined into a model of reflective practice by Abrami et al. (2009, as cited in Johnson, 2013) that considers reflection occurring in three stages:

- Planning before the performance, asking *What?*
- Doing during the performance, asking *So what?*
- Reflecting after the performance is complete, asking *Now what?*

I think the questions associated with the three phases are an excellent way to understand the complexity of reflection and to teach all aspects of the construct in a meaningful and useful manner.

Reflective practice is valuable for students, but too often done after the fact to improve *future* performance, not taking full advantage of the other aspects of reflective practice. Equally important is for students to develop their own metacognitive voices or the ability to reflect-in-action to guide performance as it is occurring. Faculty can promote this process in several ways: (a) by teaching students about reflection-in-action (or metacognition), specifically the value it has in regulating study habits, improving performance, and becoming self-regulated learners; (b) modeling their metacognitive voices by asking probing questions during online discussions or voicing the thought processes they are using to problem solve; and (c) by providing opportunities for reflection-on-action as a means of retrieval practice and self-evaluation (Brown et al., 2014; Schraw, 1998).

Deep and Surface Processing

Two other constructs have an impact on memory formation that involves the approach students take to studying and processing information—*surface* or *deep processing* and *cognitive load*. Studies reported by Beattie, Collins, and McInnes (1997) indicated that students' approach to learning was dependent on multiple factors, such as the requirements of the task, perceived amount of time to complete the task, overall workload, personal interest or engagement, locus of control or means of motivation (intrinsic vs. extrinsic), level of anxiety, and perceived relevance of the content. We have long known that the requirements of the educational environment, particularly assessment, drive learning (Beattie et al., 1997). Tulving and Thomson (1973) related this phenomenon to *encoding specificity*. Their research revealed that "encoding of target words was influenced by the list cues present at input and by the subjects' expectations that they would be tested with those cues" (p. 369).

Students use the *surface* approach to learning when their goal is memorization. Beattie et al. (1997) describe the surface approach as (a) memorizing without critical evaluation, that is, taking everything at face value; (b) focusing on facts without searching for the underlying concepts and principles; and (c) focusing on passing the test and not long-term learning. If students know they will be tested using knowledge-based multiple-choice questions (MCQs), they will study appropriately, use a surface approach, and memorize the information as unrelated tidbits to be recalled by a cue from a test question.

According to Karpicke and Grimaldi (2012), this surface approach to learning "is thought to produce poorly organized knowledge that lacks coherence and integration, which is reflected in failures to make inferences and transfer knowledge to new problems" (p. 160). Dolmans, Loyens, Marcq, and Gijbels (2015) indicated that the approach to studying is not a stable and consistent trait within students, but most likely a state in response to the requirements of the environment, such as the assessment. The type of assessment and students' metacognitive self-knowledge allows them to match their preferred study strategies for the type of task, which all too often leads to surface processing to pass a test.

The *deep* approach to learning is characterized by students making meaning out of what they read and to "relate information to prior knowledge, to structure ideas into comprehensible wholes, and to critically evaluate knowledge and conclusions presented in the text" (Dolmans et al., 2015, para. 4). The deep approach requires (a) studying to learn for understanding using a critical approach, (b) recalling prior knowledge and experience, and (c) carefully comparing presented evidence with arguments and conclusions (Beattie et al., 1997). Both metacognition and reflection are strategies that can promote deep processing.

Specific teaching methods can promote deep learning. Dolmans et al. (2015) reviewed 21 studies on problem-based learning (PBL) that studied the process of PBL with respect to the approach students used to learn—deep or surface. PBL is a case-based approach to learning that requires active, self-directed learning strategies and functions as an assessment as well as a teaching method. Not surprising, 11 of the 21 studies showed that PBL does promote deep learning with no effect on surface learning.

Transfer of Learning

Deep learning provides the foundation for transfer of learning, which is the ability to use information in different contexts, either similar or quite different from how it was learned. Multiple types of transfer have been described in the literature: lateral and vertical, literal and figural, near and far, and specific and nonspecific (Merriam & Leahy, 2005; Mestre, 2005). For our purposes, *near* and *far transfer* are most pertinent. Near transfer involves using information in a new but similar situation when compared to how it was learned. Application of what was learned in the classroom or simulation lab to actual care of a patient is a form of near transfer. This involves understanding what was taught instead of simply recalling memorized facts (Glaser, 1991). Far transfer refers to using information learned in one situation to a new and different situation (Detterman & Sternberg, 1993; Haskell, 2001; Mayer, 2002), which is really the goal of higher education (Mayer, 1998). We want our students to learn in such a way that they can take what was learned in school into the workplace in their new role and apply it to various situations and problems.

Mayer (1998) identified three prerequisites for problem-solving transfer: *skill, metaskill,* and *will. Skill* refers to the learner's ability to (a) extract salient content from a lesson, (b) make sense of this information, (c) activate existing associated knowledge, and (d) integrate the new information into what is known in a meaningful way. *Metaskill* is another term for metacognition and refers to both knowledge and regulation of cognition (thinking). This skill is essential for students to monitor their thinking as well as regulate the process. *Will* refers to the learner's motivation for learning that is tied into self-efficacy or belief in his or her own ability to perform successfully. Overall, Mayer's conceptualization of the requisites for transfer are the most complete with the addition of will, as motivation is essential for both learning and transfer.

Self-Regulated Learning

In order to learn, students must be motivated and channel that motivation into directing their learning (Miller, 2014). Zimmerman (1989) stated that "students can be described as self-regulated to the degree that they are metacognitively, motivationally, and behaviorally active participants in their own learning process" (p. 329). Note that the word *active* is used here, which is key to the process of self-regulation.

Being metacognitively active refers back to what we discussed in an earlier section, specifically employing *strategic* metacognition. Strategic metacognitive knowledge encompasses knowing about various learning strategies as well as knowledge of strategies to monitor and regulate learning.

Being motivationally active with regard to self-regulated learning refers to intrinsic motivation or "the inherent interest in and valuing of an activity" (Miller, 2014, p. 168), which depends to some degree on attitudes, level of anxiety, expectancy, and affect (Zimmerman, 1989). Continued motivation is, to some degree, based upon the perceived success from working diligently to meet goals (a behavior), and this self-satisfaction serves to sustain motivation (Zimmerman, 2002).

To be behaviorally active, students must believe in their ability to succeed if they apply themselves, set goals that are achievable, and maintain an interest in achieving the goal, as well as value learning itself (Pintrich, 2002). Being behaviorally active is a product of self-efficacy and study strategies that include effective time management, self-testing, and goal setting.

Multiple Ways of Thinking

For Benner, Sutphen, Leonard, and Day (1984/2010), the term *critical thinking* was thought to be too restrictive, especially when considering the complexity of today's clinical nursing practice. They referred to the term critical thinking as a "catch all phrase for the many forms of thinking that nurses use in practice" (p. 84). Additional terms to be considered are *clinical reasoning, diagnostic reasoning, clinical reasoning-in-transition, clinical imagination, creative reasoning, scientific reasoning,* and *format criterial reasoning.* The point Benner and colleagues are trying to make, I believe, is that the "multiple ways of thinking" (p. 85) required of nurses differs and is dependent upon the *type* of nursing practice and as of yet has not been assigned a satisfactory term to adequately describe the complex and inclusive process. Nevertheless, we, as educators, are required to prepare our students for the type of thinking required in practice. To achieve this, we must teach content within the same context in which it will be encountered in the specific nursing roles our students aspire to and are studying for. Doing so will help them build rich mental models that are well cued for easy retrieval when they encounter a similar situation in practice.

So What?

So why is all of this important? The goal of education is transfer. In order for that to occur, deep learning should be promoted using authentic teaching methods so that rich mental models with multiple cues for retrieval are created. Understanding how we learn and the specific concepts related to learning are important for educators, especially when teaching online. If we understand that new mental models are created when the learner encounters unfamiliar information or existing mental models are built upon when newly encountered information adds to or modifies existing knowledge, the value of activating prior knowledge before the learner engages with new material makes sense. Faculty can control cognitive load, to some degree, by strategically choosing teaching methods appropriate to the online environment, being mindful that the complexity of instructional elements matches the learning level of the students, and intuitively organizing the LMS so that it is not in the way of learning. When we model our problem-solving processes during discussions by making our metacognitive thought processes explicit, students will quickly learn the value of metacognition or reflection-in-action and begin to ask themselves and others more probing questions. In addition, instructors should choose assessments that will ultimately drive learning in the desired direction so as to promote deep learning, which will then more readily transfer to the workplace.

LEARNING AND ASSESSMENT

The value assessments hold as additional teaching strategies has not been maximized in nursing education, which is largely due to the timing of assessments during a course and the overemphasis on summative assessment. Multiple-choice tests are typically scheduled at midterm and the end of the course to assess learning with little time available for test review, which is a valuable way for students to learn from what they answered correctly (validate learning) or from their mistakes (formative assessment).

Faculty's perceived need to *cover* ever-expanding content also impacts time available for test review. This results in faculty setting aside office hours to review tests on an individual student basis, which is not only an inefficient approach, but one that takes even more of faculty's precious time.

Another concern with reviewing a test with the entire class is test integrity and the ability to reuse test questions in future classes, which leaves faculty with a dilemma as to the best course of action. Although this is a realistic concern, it relates back to the timing of assessments and the overemphasis on one single test—or two if the final test is cumulative—to assess whether students have learned the content. This will be discussed in more detail later in this chapter in the section From Cognitive Science Research. At this juncture, understanding the difference between formative and summative assessments is important in order to begin to grasp how assessments can be used as teaching methods.

Formative Assessment

Formative assessment has been described as assessment *for* learning or feedback that promotes learning (Kennedy, Chan, Fok, & Yu, 2008). By definition, formative assessment is not connected to termination of an educational activity or a final grade, as it takes place as part of the process of learning (Gikandi, Morrow, & Davis, 2011). Formative assessment comes from feedback from faculty with the goal of helping students improve their work through reflection, reconsideration of their perspectives, and review of educational resources (Sadler, 1989).

Recognizing the need for formative assessment often occurs during small group discussions, for example, when faculty discover that a student is struggling to understand the content and apply it to the question at hand. In other words, faculty recognize that the student has reached his or her zone of proximal development (ZPD), or his or her current ability without assistance, a concept discussed in greater detail in Chapter 2. So, from the learning perspective of formative assessment, faculty have recognized that the student is struggling to learn. From an assessment perspective, faculty have assessed what the student seems to know and understand and has made a mental note of the student's ability *at that particular point in time*. By reading the student's subsequent posts on the ongoing discussion, assessment continues as faculty determine if their intervention was sufficient to promote understanding at the necessary level to successfully complete the task and meet the objectives. Thus, formative assessment has two sides, an *assessment* side and a *teaching* side, which occur simultaneously.

Summative Assessment

Summative assessment, an assessment *of* learning (Kennedy et al., 2008) quantitatively, evaluates performance in the form of a grade that indicates to the learner and other stakeholders at what level the student has learned and met the identified learning outcomes of the assignment (Sadler, 1989). However, summative assessment can also become a means of teaching and learning, if the activity is well placed in the course. By that I mean time exists for continued dialogue with students after they receive a grade. For example, small group discussions are used for formative and summative assessments. If faculty have provided adequate facilitation throughout the discussion, most students will have met the desired learning outcomes.

Another Perspective

Summative assessment is, from my perspective, an *unnecessary evil* in higher education designed to sort students. Some pass, some fail, but they are all assigned a grade to indicate the level at which they performed. Online discussions are typically graded and become part of the final grade for the course, often encompassing a fair percentage of that grade. After all, they are the main learning space in the course and vital, I might add, to transforming nursing education by addressing the recommendations of Benner and colleagues (1984/2010) to "teach for a sense of salience, situated cognition, and action in particular situations" (p. 82), integrate *knowing that* with *knowing how* and *knowing when*, emphasize multiple ways of thinking, and promote formation into the role. Although small group discussions are likened to classroom discussion, there is really no comparison. Students *choose* to participate in a classroom discussion, whereas students online *must* participate, as a fair percentage of their grade—enough to fail the course—is attached to participation that contributes to the ongoing dialogue.

Faculty's job—and this is important—is to create a discussion topic that is engaging and relevant, and to be present in the discussion to guide learning to meet the desired outcomes. So, my point in all of this is that if we do our job, summative assessment should be fairly straightforward for faculty, and the assigned grade not unexpected for students. Summative assessment would simply involve assigning a grade based on objective criteria in the discussion rubric and commenting on how the student could improve future performance if this is not clear from the rubric itself. Including a few encouraging words is always appreciated by students. Additional comments that pertain to the procedural side of discussions, such as posting on time, replying to the required number of classmates' posts, and adhering to the word limit on the posts, if not specified in the rubric, are appropriate as they would impact performance in future discussions. I do not see the need for faculty to provide detailed feedback pertaining to a lack of knowledge, understanding, or application that the *student can do nothing to remedy*. The discussion is over. Consider that if student learning is at the heart of the faculty role, evidence exists that students are engaged and applying themselves in the discussions, and, if adequate feedback and direct instruction have been provided during the discussion, I question the need to deduct points. My concern is that faculty are comparing students' performance with each other and not against objective criteria. Discussing the difference between norm-referenced and criterion-referenced grading will be useful at this juncture.

Norm-Referenced and Criterion-Referenced Grading

In order for grading to occur, a standard or criteria must be available for comparison against the student's performance. In days gone by, when high-stakes testing was used for sorting students—to determine those who were suitable for college, those for whom a trade was a good choice, or ordering students to provide a class rank—norm-referenced testing ruled. Student's performance was compared to other student's performance, with higher performing students setting the bar. According to Glaser (1963):

> Such measures need provide little or no information . . . in terms of what the individual can do. They tell that one student is more or less proficient than another, but do not tell how proficient either of them is with respect to the subject matter tasks involved. (p. 520)

Unfortunately, even today faculty compare one student's performance to another's, but in a much less formal and often unconscious way. Well-performing students set the standard for comparison instead of comparing performance against a standard, such as criteria in a rubric.

Criterion-referenced grading, on the other hand, compares student's performance to a predetermined set of criteria, typically a rubric, where performance is on a continuum from none to desired performance. When a rubric is used for grading, the criteria are objectively stated and the student's performance compared with those criteria. This serves to keep faculty focused on the criteria and eliminates comparisons of performance with other students (Glaser, 1963).

Because nursing students must master the content (*knowing*) as well as the skills of using this content in practice (*doing*) to function in the complexity that is nursing practice, comparing them to another student will not serve them in their future role. Their performance must be assessed as compared to known competencies that are needed for the role. By providing ongoing formative feedback using scaffolding to promote learning, students will be guided toward *uncovering* what faculty want them to in order to learn deeply and meet the objective of the course. If this happens as the discussion unfolds, no surprises will occur when the discussion has ended and a grade assigned.

FROM COGNITIVE SCIENCE RESEARCH

The Testing Effect and Spaced Study

One would think that cognitive psychology research pertaining to how people learn would be readily put to practice in schools, but as Pashler, Rohrer, Cepeda, and Carpenter (2007) lament, this is not the case, especially in regard to assessment practices. In particular, testing continues to be timed at midterm and the end of a course as summative assessment when compelling research indicates that frequent quizzes used as formative assessment improve long-term learning, retention, retrieval, and transfer

(Roediger & Karpicke, 2006). This phenomenon—termed the *testing effect* or *retrieval practice effect*—refers to "the research finding that testing does not just measures [sic] knowledge, but also alters the learning process itself so that new knowledge is retained and transferred more effectively" (Kerfoot et al., 2010, p. 332). Multiple studies have shown that taking a test has a greater effect on future retention and recall of that material than simply studying the material repeatedly or highlighting passages (Roediger, 2013). In effect, test taking affords valuable practice *retrieving* what was learned and strengthens the *process* of doing so (Roediger & Karpicke, 2006).

Frequent testing encourages students to engage in *spaced study* as opposed to *massed study*. When students know they will be tested weekly, they are more apt to complete the readings and study at the time the content is assigned (spaced study), rather than procrastinating until just before the midterm or final exam (massed study or cramming) (Carpenter, 2012). Kerfoot et al. (2010) define spaced study as "the psychological research finding that information is learned and retained more effectively when presented and repeated during spaced intervals of time (spaced distribution)" (p. 331). Although this seems like a choice students make in their study habits, course design can influence these habits.

The research on spaced study is based on what is termed a *study–no study* pattern involving study episodes interspersed with time away from studying. In cognitive psychology terms, this means two study episodes are separated by an interstudy interval (ISI), or a period of no study, lasting from a few minutes to days. The second study episode is followed by another no-study period, called the *retention interval* (RI), which occurs prior to taking the test (Pashler et al., 2007). So, the sequence is basically study, wait, study again, rest, and take the test. A number of studies were done in which the duration of time varied in the ISI and between the RI and test taking to evaluate the process of rather short-term learning, as well as long-term retention of professional skills (Kerfoot, 2009; Kerfoot et al., 2010; Pashler et al., 2007). Overall, these studies focused on the learning of *basic* facts, skills, concepts, and procedures, or the lower cognitive skills of memorization and understanding. Testing was done with questions that involved recall (retrieval from memory or fill in the blank) or recognition (multiple-choice). The results of a study involving urology residents indicated that spaced study using board preparation-style questions increased retention for up to 2 years (Kerfoot, 2009). Pashler et al. (2007) learned from their research that the positive effects of spaced education on declarative knowledge were as follows:

- Feedback provided on incorrect answers on a fact-based test afforded a fivefold increase in accurate recall on the final test.
- Feedback delayed 24 hours improved recall.

- Matching retrieval practice to how facts will be later retrieved in the workplace improves recall even if the practice of doing so is covert (not verbalized).
- Testing lessened forgetting when compared to restudying the content.

Kapler, Weston, and Wiseheart (2015) conducted a study with undergraduate students who were divided into two groups. One group reviewed the lecture material 1 day after the lecture and the other group completed their review 8 days after the lecture. Both groups then took a test 5 weeks later that comprised both *knowledge-* and *application-*level questions. Students whose study was separated by 8 days scored higher on both levels of questions, underscoring the value of greater spacing of study. Of note is that application-level questions, considered on a higher cognitive level and possibly questions requiring transfer of previously learned concepts to a new situation, were included in the study. This has implications for complex learning that goes beyond remembering or recalling.

For retention of material and long-term learning, the results across the board from various studies indicated that testing just minutes after the second study episode without an RI produced better *recall,* but poorer long-term *retrieval,* which perhaps explains why massed study (cramming) may result in an acceptable performance on a test, but faster forgetting. As the goal of teaching is for students to learn deeply in order to recall (retrieve) the information when needed in practice and to be able to think flexibly to transfer what was learned to their future role, spaced study should be encouraged and the benefits of the testing effect employed. The best way to accomplish both is to quiz students frequently, provide correct answers for incorrect responses, and delay feedback on incorrect answers 24 hours. Based on their research, Roediger and Pyc (2012) believed that spaced practice and the testing effect, when used consistently, would certainly improve the learning of basic facts and concepts, providing a foundation for deeper learning in the future. If summative tests are part of the course design, questions should be similar, if not the same, as those on the formative tests.

Variables of the Testing Effect

Type of Test

Roediger and Karpicke (2006) found that the testing effect was stronger with recall (or generative) questions, such as fill in the blank and short answer, compared with MCQs requiring recognition of the right answer. Nevertheless, taking a multiple-choice test did demonstrate improved recall over restudying the material. The authors did caution that the research was not consistent in this regard and additional investigation is warranted with regard to multiple-choice tests. However, given that the software in most LMSs can automatically grade MCQs and provide feedback to students, this type of test is more efficient than fill in the blank or short answer, which faculty must grade by hand. In courses or programs in which summative testing is not used, the research is telling us that frequent multiple-choice tests used as formative assessment will be more effective in promoting retrieval than repeated studying. What also seems promising is that if students can take these tests multiple times to learn the material, their studying will be spaced, which will improve long-term retention.

The Role of Feedback on Tests

Research on feedback is relevant here (Pashler et al., 2007). Surprisingly, *immediate* feedback on incorrect answers was not superior in promoting retention when compared to delayed feedback—another less-than-intuitive research finding. In fact, delayed feedback for incorrect answers actually improved retention. The reason for this may be related to the spaced study effect of revisiting the content at a later date. Of interest is that without feedback, a phenomenon called the *negative suggestion effect* can occur with multiple-choice and true–false questions. That is, over time students may recall incorrect answers they gave to test questions and mistakenly think they were the right answers. This issue worsens as more distractors are added to the questions. However, feedback delayed for 24 hours on questions answered incorrectly eliminates this issue (Roediger & Karpicke, 2006).

With regard to quizzes given online, feedback can be easily added to the distractors (incorrect answers) on MCQs in the LMS. To delay feedback, faculty can set a date in the software so that students must wait at least 24 hours after the test closes to review the answers. As online quizzes should be open for at least 5 days so that students can arrange time to take them, this is a reasonable approach that also serves to alleviate potential cheating. If the correct answers are not validated until after the test closes, sharing answers with other students who have yet to take the quiz cannot be done with confidence.

Spaced Education: An Innovation in Teaching

Kerfoot et al. (2010) created an educational strategy called *SpacedEd*, which was offered online for a number of years and that offered lessons on a wide variety of topics. I had the opportunity to not only participate in one of these modules (cardiac pathology), but also to use a module on basic physical assessment content during an advanced health assessment course with graduate doctor of nursing practice (DNP) students. After signing up for a course, an MCQ was sent via e-mail daily with a link that directed the learner to answer the question online. Feedback was provided for both incorrect and correct answers with links included for remediation or continued study. Each test included approximately 30 to 35 questions. Any question that the learner answered incorrectly was resent intermittently until answered correctly, thus spacing and interleaving the questions. Questions that students answered correctly were also revisited, but at longer intervals. This cycle continued until all of the questions were answered correctly. Kerfoot et al. (2010) conducted a study involving urology residents that compared bolus delivery of questions (all at once) with spaced delivery. Although the bolus delivery resulted in increased recall after 3 months, recall then fell off. However, for the spaced delivery group, retention and recall persisted to 7 months when the study ended.

Interleaving

Interleaving is an instructional strategy that is best explained by comparing it to massed practice, or blocked practice as it is also called. Massed practice involves studying one bit of content over and over until it is mastered (or memorized). Cramming for a test is considered massed practice. Interleaved practice involves mixing up content, but revisiting each part at intervals. Blocked practice would be depicted by AAAABBBBCCCC, and interleaved study by ABCABCABC (Pan, 2015, para. 2). Massed practice often results in improved performance immediately after studying, which is why the results of cramming for a test the next day often pan out. However, this type of study results in rapid forgetting. Interleaving practice seems very counterintuitive and students often find it more effortful. However, it results in better long-term learning than massed practice (Brown et al., 2014).

LEARNING-STYLE INVENTORIES

The original intent of learning-style inventories was for *students* to understand how they learn best (Fleming & Mills, 1992; Oermann, 2013). Reading the nursing literature on learning styles, the take-away is that knowing students' preferred learning style is necessary in order to choose appropriate teaching methods to appeal to all learners in the class. Thus, learners learn best when their preferred style is used as the teaching method (Brown et al., 2014). This is an enormous, if not improbable, task for faculty. In the online environment, which is primarily text-based, recorded mini-lectures and podcasts can be used. However, overall teaching methods are limited in this modality.

The topic of learning styles is wrought with controversy. Studies on learning styles seem to be divided into two camps: those who promote educational strategies matching learning styles to maximize learning, and those who feel that deliberately mismatching learning styles will increase the variety of ways in which a student can approach learning (Jeffrey, 2008). The construct of learning styles is imprecise and encompasses, according to Cassidy (2004), "a variety of definitions, theoretical positions, models, interpretations, and measures of the construct" (p. 420). Pashler, McDaniel, Rohrer, and Bjork (2008) reviewed the literature on learning-style inventories and found no well-designed study that demonstrated the validity of these instruments to assess learning styles. They concluded that the widespread use of these inventories in education is simply not supported.

IMPLICATIONS FOR COURSE DESIGN

The information presented so far has implication for course design, which is discussed in subsequent chapters. When cases include a problem built into a context applicable to the student's future role, the student is asked to problem solve—an activity the brain was designed to do from an evolutionary perspective. In order for the student to solve the problem, memorization will not help. Deep processing of information is required as students read, synthesize, and apply what they have read to the case. In addition, the context supports the creation of multiple cues for retrieval, and frequent retrieval deepens learning and creates additional cues for retrieval. By storing the information as a case in cognitive structures, the information has been stored in the same manner in which it will be retrieved when the student encounters a similar problem in the workplace.

Frequent formative testing of the low-stakes variety (few points attached) can serve several purposes—activating prior knowledge, promoting transfer, and strengthening memory traces by practicing retrieval of newly learned information. Test taking is a more efficient way for students to learn compared to spending time rereading and highlighting information. Although this approach seems less than intuitive, surprisingly, students do not object to frequent quizzes, instead finding them beneficial to learning (Roediger & Karpicke, 2006).

THE TAKE-AWAY

Who our learners are, how they learn and at what level, and the strategies available to help them learn more deeply have implications for course design. The terms defined and discussed in this chapter combined with the educational theories and concepts presented in Chapter 2 should provide a sound foundation for the chapters that follow as well as online course design.

REFERENCES

American Association of Colleges of Nursing. (2014). *Building a framework for the future: Advancing higher education in nursing.* Washington, DC: Author.

Atkinson, R. C., & Shiffrin, R. M. (1968). Human memory: A proposed system and its control processes. *Psychology of Learning and Motivation, 2,* 89–195.

Beattie, V., Collins, B., & McInnes, B. (1997). Deep and surface learning: A simple or simplistic dichotomy? *Accounting Education, 6*(1), 1–12.

Benner, P. (1984/2001). *From novice to expert: Excellence and power in clinical nursing practice.* Upper Saddle River, NJ: Prentice Hall Health. (Commemorative edition. Original work published 1984.)

Benner, P., Sutphen, M., Leonard, V., & Day, L. (1984/2010). *Educating nurses: A call for radical transformation.* San Francisco, CA: Jossey-Bass.

Boud, D. (2001). Using journal writing to enhance reflective practice. *New Directions for Adult and Continuing Education, 90,* 9–17.

Brown, P. C., Roediger, H. L., III, & McDaniel, M. A. (2014). *Make it stick: The science of successful learning.* Cambridge, MA: Belknap Press.

Carpenter, S. K. (2012). Testing enhances the transfer of learning. *Current Directions in Psychological Science, 21*(5), 279–283.

Cassidy, S. (2004). Learning styles: An overview of theories, models, and methods. *Educational Psychology, 24*(4), 419–444.

Chung, E., Turnbull, D., & Chur-Hansen, A. (2014). Who are "non-traditional students"? A systematic review of published definitions in research on mental health or tertiary students. *Educational Research and Reviews, 9*(23), 1224–1238.

Detterman, D. K., & Sternberg, R. J. (Eds.). (1993). *Transfer on trial: Intelligence, cognition, and instruction.* Norwood, NJ: Ablex.

Dolmans, D. H., Loyens, S. M., Marcq, H., & Gijbels, D. (2015). Deep and surface learning in problem-based learning: A review of the literature. *Advances in Health Sciences Education, 21*(5), 1087–1112. Retrieved from http://link.springer.com/article/10.1007/s10459-015-9645-6

Flavell, J. H. (1979). Metacognition and cognitive monitoring: A new area of cognitive-developmental inquiry. *American Psychologist, 34*(10), 906–911.

Fleming, N. D., & Mills, C. (1992). Not another inventory, rather a catalyst for reflection. *Improve the Academy, 11,* 137–146.

Gikandi, J. W., Morrow, D., & Davis, N. E. (2011). Online formative assessment in higher education: A review of the literature. *Computers & Education, 57,* 2333–2351.

Glaser, R. (1963). Instructional technology and the measurement of learning outcomes: Some questions. *American Psychologist, 18*(7), 519–521.

Glaser, R. (1991). The maturing of the relationship between the science of learning and cognition and educational practice. *Learning and Instruction, 1,* 129–144.

Haskell, R. E. (2001). *Transfer of learning: Cognition, instruction, and reasoning.* San Diego, CA: Academic Press.

Jeffrey, L. M. (2008). Learning orientations: Diversity in higher education. *Learning and Individual Differences, 19*, 195–208.

Johnson, J. A. (2013). Reflective learning, reflective practice, and metacognition. *Journal for Nurses in Professional Development, 29*(1), 46–48.

Kapler, I. V., Weston, T., & Wiseheart, M. (2015). Spacing in a simulated undergraduate classroom: Long-term benefits for factual and higher-level learning. *Learning and Instruction, 36*, 38–45.

Karpicke, J. D., & Grimaldi, P. J. (2012). Retrieval-based learning: A perspective for enhancing meaningful learning. *Educational Psychological Review, 24*, 401–418.

Kennedy, K. J., Chan, J. K. S., Fok, P. K., & Yu, W. M. (2008). Forms of assessment and their potential for enhancing learning: Conceptual and cultural issues. *Educational Research for Policy and Practice, 7*(3), 197–207.

Kerfoot, B. P. (2009). Learning benefits of on-line spaced education persist for 2 years. *Journal of Urology, 181*, 2671–2673.

Kerfoot, B. P., Fu, Y., Baker, H., Connelly, D., Ritchey, M. L., & Genega, E. M. (2010). Online spaced education generates transfer and improves long-term retention of diagnostic skills: A randomized controlled trial. *Journal of the American College of Surgeons, 211*(3), 331–337.

Mann, K., Gordon, J., & MacLeod, A. (2009). Reflection and reflective practice in health professions education: A systematic review. *Advances in Health Science Education, 14*, 595–621.

Mayer, R. E. (1998). Cognitive, metacognitive, and motivational aspects of problem solving. *Instructional Science, 26*, 49–63.

Mayer, R. E. (2002). Rote versus meaningful learning. *Theory Into Practice, 41*(4), 226–232.

Merriam, S. B., & Leahy, B. (2005). Learning transfer: A review of the research in adult education and training. *PAACE Journal of Lifelong Learning, 14*, 1–24.

Mestre, J. P. (Ed.). (2005). *Transfer of learning from a modern multidisciplinary perspective.* Greenwich, CT: Information Age Publishing.

Miller, M. D. (2014) *Minds online: Teaching effectively with technology.* Cambridge, MA: Harvard University Press.

Nairne, J. S., Thompson, S. R., & Pandeirada, N. S. (2007). Adaptive memory: Survival processing enhances retention. *Journal of Experimental Psycholgy, 33*(2), 263–273.

National Council of State Boards of Nursing. (2013). National Nursing Workforce Survey. Retrieved from https://www.ncsbn.org/workforce.htm

Oermann, M. H. (2013). *Teaching in nursing and role of the educator: The complete guide to practice in teaching, evaluation and curriculum development.* New York, NY: Springer Publishing.

Pan, S. C. (2015, August 4). The interleaving effect: Mixing it up boosts learning: Studying related skills or concepts in parallel is a surprisingly effective way to train your brain. *Scientific American.* Retrieved from http://www.scientificamerican.com/article/the-interleaving-effect-mixing-it-up-boosts-learning

Pashler, H., McDaniel, M., Rohrer, D., & Bjork, R. (2008). Learning styles: Concepts and evidence. *Psychological Science in the Public Interest, 9*(3), 105–119.

Pashler, H., Rohrer, D., Cepeda, N. J., & Carpenter, S. K. (2007). Enhancing learning and retarding forgetting: Choices and consequences. *Psychonomic Bulletin & Review, 14*(2), 187–193.

Pintrich, P. (2002). The role of metacognitive knowledge in learning, teaching, and assessing. *Theory Into Practice, 41*(4), 219–225.

Radford, A. W., Cominole, M., & Skomsvold, P. (2015). Web tables: Demographic and enrollment characteristics of nontraditional undergraduates, 2011–12. U.S. Department of Education. Retrieved from https://nces.ed.gov/pubs2015/2015025.pdf

Reese, A. C. (1998). Implications of results from cognitive science research for medical education. *Medical Education Online, 3*(1), 1–9. Retrieved from http://www.med-ed-online.org/f0000010.htm

Roediger, H. L. (2013). Applying cognitive psychology to education: Translational educational science. *Psychological Science in the Public Interest, 14*(1) 1–3.

Roediger, H. L., & Karpicke, J. D. (2006). The power of testing memory: Basic research and implications for educational practice. *Perspectives on Psychological Science, 1*(3), 181–210.

Roediger, H. L., & Pyc, M. A. (2012). Applying cognitive psychology to education: Complexities and prospects. *Journal of Applied Research in Memory and Cognition, 1*, 263–265.

Rosen, L. D. (2011). Teaching the iGeneration. *Educational Leadership, 68*(5), 10–15. Retrieved from http://www.ascd.org/publications/educational-leadership/feb11/vol68/num05/Teaching-the-iGeneration.aspx

Ross-Gordon, J. M. (2011). Research on adult learners: Supporting the needs of a student population that is no longer nontraditional. *Peer Review, 13*(1). Retrieved from https://www.aacu.org/publications-research/periodicals/research-adult-learners-supporting-needs-student-population-no

Sadler, D. R. (1989). Formative assessment and the design of instructional systems. *Instructional Science, 18*, 119–144.

Schön, D. (1983). *The reflective practitioner.* San Francisco, CA: Jossey-Bass.

Schraw, G. (1998). Promoting general metacognitive awareness. *Instructional Science, 26*, 113–125.

Sweller, J., Van Merrienboer, J. J., & Paas, F. G. (1998). Cognitive architecture and instructional design. *Educational Psychology Review, 10*(3), 251–296.

Tulving, E., & Thomson, D. M. (1973). Encoding specificity and retrieval processes in episodic memory. *Psychological Review, 80*(5), 352–373.

Weinstein, C. E., & Mayer, R. E. (1983). The teaching of learning strategies. *Innovation Abstracts, 5*(32). Retrieved from http://files.eric.ed.gov/fulltext/ED237180.pdf

Wilson, J. L. (2002). Generation X: Who are they? What do they want? *NEA Higher Education Journal.* Retrieved from http://www.nea.org/assets/img/PubThoughtAndAction/TAA_98Fal_02.pdf

Young, J. Q., Van Merrienboer, J., Durning, S., & Ten Cate, O. (2014). Cognitive load theory: Implications for medication education: AMEE Guide No. 86. *Medical Teacher, 36*(5), 371–384.

Zimmerman, B. J. (1989). A social cognitive view of self-regulated academic learning. *Journal of Educational Psychology, 81*, 329–339.

Zimmerman, B. J. (2002). Becoming a self-regulated learner: An overview. *Theory Into Practice, 41*(2), 64–70.

2

Concepts and Theories to Support Teaching and Learning

I would imagine that most of today's faculty have spent countless hours sitting in classrooms taking notes as the teacher lectured. This was the teaching method du jour for decades. Online education has provided an opportunity to change that. However, we cannot simply upload our lectures and call it "online education." What this change has afforded is the opportunity to combine how adults learn with appropriate teaching methods and assessment strategies to support learning. This chapter discusses adult learning theory and educational theories and models appropriate for the online environment. Combining this material with what we discussed in Chapter 1, the reader should have the necessary theoretical and practical knowledge foundational for online course development and design.

ANDRAGOGY AND PEDAGOGY

Educators have intuitively known for centuries, dating back to the time of Plato, that teaching adults is fundamentally different from teaching children (Knowles, Holton, & Swanson, 2015). According to Knowles et al. (2015), pedagogy dates back to the 12th century in religious schools in Europe. Pedagogical methods were used exclusively in public schools and higher education in 19th-century Europe and the United States until the past decade, when adult education theory became more mainstream.

Pedagogy

According to Knowles (1980), pedagogy can be defined as the "art and science of teaching children" (p. 40). Although the original leaning was that of educating children, the term continues to be used in the broader context when referring to the elements of teaching. Pedagogy is a teacher-centered and teacher-driven theory of *teaching* in which the students have a passive and dependent role in their education (McAuliffe, Hargreaves, Winter, & Chadwick, 2009). Although this approach is quite appropriate for young children, as children age and become less dependent, efforts should be made to adjust teaching methods to meet their maturation. However, many educators continued to depend on this model when teaching in higher education because it was efficient and basically the only teaching method they knew; it was the way *they* were taught.

Andragogy or Adult Learning Theory

Although the term *andragogy* was first explored in the early 19th century in Germany, it was unknown in the United States until Knowles's seminal article was published in the early 1970s (Knowles, 1973). And, although Knowles began his lifelong passion with adult education over 40 years ago, widespread discussion of the differences between educating children and educating adults, adoption of the adult learning model in higher education, and the implications for teaching and learning that arose from the assumptions of andragogy are fairly recent events.

Just as pedagogy refers to the art and science of educating children, the term andragogy refers to that of helping adults learn. It is more of a model of learning, whereas pedagogy is a model of teaching (McAuliffe et al., 2009). Knowles concept of andragogy was based on a set of assumptions that grew from four to six as he refined his model over a period of 20 years (Knowles et al., 2015), which explains the disparity in the number of assumptions published during this time and even after (Forrest & Peterson, 2006; McAuliffe et al., 2009; Merriam, 2001). The assumptions of andragogy and pedagogy emanate from six related constructs, namely, "(a) the learner's need to know, (b) self-concept of the learner, (c) prior experience of the learner, (d) readiness to learn, (e) orientation to learning, and (f) motivation to learn" (Knowles et al., 2015, pp. 4–5).

In terms of the assumptions of andragogy, the adult learner is one (a) whose need to know is driven by personal goals; (b) who has an independent self-concept and is self-directed; (c) who brings a variety of experiences to the educational setting; (d) whose identified need to learn is based on changing social roles; (e) whose learning is focused on problem solving; and (f) who is intrinsically motivated for the most part, although increased earning potential may be part of the reason for returning to school.

Criticism of the descriptions of pedagogy and andragogy has focused on whether these two constructs were antithetical, as originally conceived by Knowles, or at opposite ends of a continuum of learning, as he later came to understand (Merriam, 2001). As Norman (1999) so adroitly surmised, the difference between andragogy and pedagogy must be made on the basis of either nature or nurture, that is, mental development versus sociological phenomenon. Thus, allowing these assumptions to drive course design without question may prove problematic. Unfamiliarity with course content, limited professional experience, and well-ingrained generational characteristics, such as millennials expecting helicopter professors (Fang, 2015) to perform just like their helicopter parents, can drive an adult to be less self-directed and more dependent on the teacher for guidance and support (Knowles et al., 2015). So instead of defining the approach to teaching along dimensions of age and experience, evaluating each learning situation from the perspective of newness and complexity of content and of learners' prior experience would be more prudent.

Nursing education, especially at the RN to bachelor of science in nursing (BSN) and graduate levels, involves a heterogeneous group of students who, although they have the same basic nursing background, differ in not only their types of experience, but also the depth and breadth of that experience. Faculty cannot expect nurses with primarily a home health nursing background to share the same experience as those with critical care experience. They may even approach problem solving differently. Consequently, although adults in every sense of the word, their ability to be self-directed, goal-oriented, problem-centered, and intrinsically motivated as they return to school after many years may be accompanied by anxiety, requiring awareness and flexibility on the part of faculty.

However, one of the benefits of online education, a text-based medium, is that most of the learning occurs in small group discussions in which all students must participate. Because the majority of students are motivated to learn and are self-directed problem solvers, they are able to combine experience with the new content being taught and participate at a high level in the discussions. When students' posts in the discussions are not where they should be, and this is easily recognizable, faculty must discover why. Various strategies to assess this are discussed in detail in Chapter 11, but one cause may be that the student's zone of proximal development (ZPD) has been entered.

THE ZPD

What lies between the student's current *ability* and what awaits to be awakened to define his or her *capability* lies in the ZPD, a term that is often misunderstood. Although Vygotsky developed the concept of the ZPD in discussing the development and maturation of children, I think it applies to adults as well. When students struggle to learn, it is because the end of their knowledge, experience, and ability to understand the content *on their own* has been reached; they are stuck. This does not mean that they have not done the assigned readings or have not worked diligently to understand. It means their *ability* to figure it out on their own has reached its limits. However, their *capacity* to figure it out and learn has yet to be realized. Thus, two developmental levels must be identified: the student's actual developmental level and the ZPD (Vygotsky, 1978). In other words, the *actual developmental level* describes the *current ability* that children have or what they are able to demonstrate without help. The involvement of someone with more knowledge and experience, such as a teacher, is needed to unmask their ZPD. Thus, the ZPD is a moving target, so to speak. According to Vygotsky (1978), "what is in the zone of proximal development today will be the actual developmental level tomorrow—that is what the child can do with assistance today she will be able to do by herself tomorrow" (p. 87).

The interaction with a more knowledgeable teacher, parent, or child identifies the boundaries of the ZPD, and it is through this interaction that the child's abilities manifest. Vygotsky's (1978) perspective is that once the children come into contact with more experienced individuals, this observed higher cognitive functioning is internalized as "they grow into the intellectual life of those around them" (p. 88). Thus, learning is social before it becomes personal. However, although the process occurs within the child, the other person benefits as well, as the old saying goes—the best way to learn is to teach.

The reason Vygotsky's (1978) work is often misunderstood is that it has been inextricably linked with the facilitative process of *scaffolding* (Tudge & Scrimsher, 2003). However, Wood, Bruner, and Ross (1976), who first introduced the concept of scaffolding into the educational literature in the mid-1970s, did so 42 years after Vygotsky's death. Nevertheless, you rarely hear ZDP discussed without the term scaffolding being mentioned as necessary in order for learning to occur. Vygotsky's perspective was that a more knowledgeable individual was required to be involved without specifying the methods used to instruct. The impact of associating scaffolding with the ZPD shifted the focus from what was occurring within the child (learning) to that of what the teacher was doing (teaching), as if the active teaching itself caused the student's expanded cognitive ability, which was not Vygotsky's original intent. His intent was that in order for the learner to realize his or her capabilities, teaching must be aimed *above* the child's actual developmental ability (or what the child was currently capable of) in order to move him or her through the ZPD, which was a radical shift in educational practices from what was occurring at the time. His perspective was that "the only good learning is that which is in advance of development" (Vygotsky, 1978, p. 89).

So, is the ZPD operational for adults? I believe it is. Although the developmental process is complete, from cognitive science research as discussed in Chapter 1, the brain's ability to learn is endless—adults do continue to develop their cognitive abilities. However, understanding the ZPD, it seems that the potential ability or capability exists; one just needs the right information, direction, or guidance of someone more knowledgeable to move forward.

Recognizing that the student is stuck and cannot proceed without faculty intervention is a skill you will develop the more you teach online. Chapter 11 includes tips on how to recognize when the ZPD has been entered and your support is needed. Interestingly, in the online environment, scaffolding is an often-used facilitative skill to provide the needed support. However, many other options are available such as providing missing links through direct teaching or helping the student connect what is being learned to prior knowledge by asking pointed questions. Whatever the appropriate strategy, this is an opportunity to *customize* teaching to meet the student's unique learning needs. So, whether you take advantage of the "teachable moment" or use facilitative techniques to guide the student's thinking, the result will help to move the student through his or her ZPD and forward toward meeting the learning outcomes.

EDUCATIONAL THEORIES AND MODELS

We want to support the continued development of adult learners identified through Knowles's assumptions of andragogy such as motivated, self-directed, experienced, problem-oriented, active learners with a need to know that is goal-driven (Merriam, 2001). What will help us do so are specific theories of teaching and learning as well as a variety of interrelated concepts that are important to understand when designing online courses and teaching adults. Constructivism and social constructivism are the predominant teaching theories that support the constructs of andragogy. However, many others that exist can guide educators and are worth mention. Based on these teaching theories and the nature of teaching adults, specific teaching methods and course design are indicated. The next few sections in this chapter address pertinent theories and concepts that you will encounter in the chapters that follow.

Behaviorism

In the first half of the 20th century, instruction was embroiled in the behaviorist movement in which a stimulus in the form of a question was posed, a response was expected, and learners received positive reinforcement for correct answers. Out of this approach arose behavioral objectives, simple-to-complex sequencing of instruction, direct teaching strategies, drill-and-practice exercises, behavior modification (Mayer, 1999; Reynolds, Sinatra, & Jetton, 1996), and perhaps the notion that repeated study is what solidified learning.

The outcome of behaviorist teaching methods was learning the right answer, leaving little room for critical thinking and multiple perspectives. Unable to explain higher order cognitive functioning, behaviorism fell out of favor and the *cognitive revolution* began (Bargh & Ferguson, 2000), shifting the focus from behavior to the mind.

Cognitivism

Cognitivism gained popularity because it focused on learning via information, an opposite approach from behaviorism. According to Mayer (1999), cognitivism was based on knowledge acquisition that occurred in the mind of the learner and focused on storage of this information in long-term memory. The learner was essentially passive and the role of the educator was one of actively organizing information to present to the learner via lecture, textbook readings, and multimedia. Learning was *acquired* (Reynolds et al., 1996).

Constructivism

According to Mayer (1999), "constructivist learning occurs when learners actively create their own knowledge by trying to make sense out of material that is presented to them" (p. 143). Thus, constructivist learning requires the learner to be cognitively active, attend to relevant information, organize that information into mental models, and integrate these mental models with existing knowledge (Mayer, 1999). Savery and Duffy (1995) delineated three propositions as the foundation for their philosophic view of the constructivist teaching and learning method of problem-based learning, which is done in small discussion groups. First, the acquisition of knowledge does not occur without the learner's active involvement. Understanding requires an interaction between the learner's active cognitive processes and goals, the content, and the context. Second, cognitive dissonance or conflict drives learning, and its resolution becomes the goal. This goal-oriented behavior determines the focus of learning, helps the learner identify relevant existing knowledge, and focuses learning on what specific information deserves attention. Third, discussing ideas in the social environment collaboratively in groups tests and validates understanding and promotes elaboration of knowledge. Alternative views can be the source of cognitive dissonance, which becomes the impetus for the reorganization of knowledge and ultimately for learning (Savery & Duffy, 1995).

Social Theories of Learning

Vygotsky's work with children and his description of the ZPD introduced the role that interpersonal relationships played in learning (Vygotsky, 1978) and led to our understanding of social constructivism. However, other social theories have guided educational practices such as the Japanese concept of *ba* (Nonaka & Konno, 1998), Lave and Wenger's (1991) communities of practice, situated cognition (Brown, Collins, & Duguid, 1989), and cognitive apprenticeship (Collins, Brown, & Newman, 1987). What these theories have in common is that learning is embedded in a social, cultural, and historical context, so that the tools of the trade—such as knowledge and concepts—are linked and that *knowing* cannot be separated from *doing*.

Social Constructivism

Social constructivism, first introduced by Vygotsky (1978), posited that knowledge is socially mediated through interpersonal relationships. This is evident in his work on the ZPD in which children learned from a more knowledgeable person within a social relationship. Three assumptions are inherent in social constructivism: the role of activity, context, and language (Stetsenko & Arievitch, 1997).

The first assumption is that through interaction with the world, the individual shapes his or her developmental course. Rather than being a passive, internally driven process, development occurs as a result of the individual's interaction with the world (Stetsenko & Arievitch, 1997).

The second assumption is that cognitive development is a function of cooperation with others who share the same situation or context. This assumption "emphasizes mutuality, communication, and the social embeddedness of the self and of the individual's development" (Stetsenko & Arievitch, 1997, p. 181).

The third assumption is closely related to the first and involves language. The importance of language is that it contains "the accumulated knowledge of prior generations and can be appropriated by an individual to be used as mediating tools/devices to regulate individual behavior" (Stetsenko & Arievitch, 1997, p. 161). Language is central to development and provides the tools for discourse and meaning making.

The Japanese Concept of Ba

Interestingly, the Japanese concept of *ba*, which roughly translated means "a shared space for knowledge creation," need not be a physical place, but can also be virtual or mental, or a combination of these (Nonaka & Konno, 1998). The authors explain, "knowledge is embedded in *ba* (in these shared spaces), where it is then acquired through one's own experience or reflections on the experiences of others. If knowledge is separated from *ba*, it turns into information. . . . Information resides in media and networks. It is tangible. In contrast, knowledge resides in *ba*. It is intangible" (pp. 41–42). Although this comes from an existential framework, it expresses the notion of *creating something from nothing* when that something is intangible knowledge generation (Groarke, 2009).

Situated Cognition

Situated cognition, the work of Brown and colleagues (1989), postulated that separating knowledge or *knowing that* from activities or *knowing how* embedded in an authentic context is detrimental to learning. The researchers contended that without context, learning is inert, and knowledge is just that—isolated facts. Situated cognition likens knowledge and concepts to tools. In order to use a tool effectively, one must understand the situations or conditions under which the tool can be used as well as the context for its use. "Because tools and the way they are used reflect the particular accumulated insights of communities, it is not possible to use a tool appropriately without understanding the community or culture in which it is used" (Brown et al., 1989, p. 33). Thus, learning to use the tools of knowledge and concepts requires that they be learned in context.

The five key elements of situated cognition are context, authenticity, activity and participation, community of practice, and shared or distributed cognition (Ghefaili, 2003). *Context* refers to the situation in which knowledge exists. Brown et al. (1989) used the example of teaching words to children. Language is typically learned in the context of talking, listening, and reading. However, early teaching focused on students memorizing dictionary definitions and subsequently using the words in a sentence that had little meaning to the child. This resulted in grammatical mistakes using the words. The authors explained, "words and sentences are not islands, entire unto themselves. Language use would involve an unremitting confrontation with ambiguity, polysemy, nuance, metaphor, and so forth were these not resolved with the extralinguistic help that the context of an utterance provides" (p. 32). Teaching in context is linked to the second element—authenticity.

In educational contexts *authenticity* means "coherent, natural, meaningful, and purposeful activities that represent the ordinary practices"

(Ghefaili, 2003, p. 6). Context in nursing education might include a patient's unique situation or a professional context, such as the acute care hospital, primary care setting, or the community, and will often emerge and be dictated by the particular program of study that will prepare the nurse for a new role. However, all content can be taught within context. Even facts that are thought to require memorization will be better remembered if related to the bigger picture and taught as part of a story.

Jonassen (1999) expands our understanding of authentic by defining it in terms of *activity* from a sociohistorical, constructivist perspective. Janssen wrote, "Activity structures rely on the socio-historical context of Activity Theory (Leontev, 1979), which focuses on the activities in which community members engage, the goals of those activities, the physical setting that constrains and affords certain actions, and the tools that mediate activity" (pp. 221–222).

Participation means that learning in a situated environment is an active process, in which students engage with each other, the content, and the educational materials (Ghefaili, 2003). Learning requires communicating one's ideas, engaging in discourse, reflecting, and revising one's position in view of the opinions of others. It is a dynamic process.

The *communities of practice,* the focus of Lave and Wenger's (1991) seminal work, described learning from an anthropological viewpoint, which shifts the individual's perspective from what he or she can contribute to or take away from the community for individual development, to a sense of belonging or being part of a community in which sharing thoughts and perspectives serves to provide a sense of identity and meaning to the individual. They coined the term *legitimate peripheral participation,* which describes the process of how a newcomer (novice) to the group, through observation of the more seasoned participants (experts), soon learns the vocabulary and tools of the community and moves from limited participation to a more active and meaningful role (Lave & Wenger, 1991). Again, learning cannot occur without participation.

Continued work on the communities of practice model has implications for teaching online. The successful community of practice has three dimensions (Wenger, 1998): "mutual engagement, joint enterprise, and a shared repertoire" (p. 73), referring to the relationships that are built when a group tackles an issue to coconstruct knowledge and understanding to arrive at a solution or resolution. These three dimensions are found in online discussions and the concept is further expanded upon and brought up to date by Garrison, Anderson, and Archer (1999).

The concept that knowledge is *shared* or *distributed* is a natural extension of the idea of legitimate peripheral participation within a community of practice and describes how "cognition is not to be found within the head only; rather cognition is distributed in the world among individuals, the tools, artifacts and books that they use, and the communities and practices in which they participate" (Ghefaili, 2003, p. 7). Again, shared knowledge requires active discourse within a group that shares common goals.

Cognitive Apprenticeship

Although Brown et al. (1989) felt that any *authentic* activity, when transferred to the classroom, automatically became a classroom activity and thus no longer authentic, their conceptualization of knowledge and concepts as tools led them to develop the cognitive apprenticeship model, a system that involves an expert working with novices to teach them a trade.

Cognitive apprenticeship takes on some of the same characteristics except that the goal is to achieve specific outcomes by learning complex tasks from a problem-based perspective through reasoning and collaborative problem solving with other novices. Teaching is done within the student's ZPD in that the tasks are more difficult than the student could handle independently (Ghefaili, 2003). Although this type of situated cognition is most appropriately used to learn psychomotor skills, the six teaching strategies of modeling, coaching, scaffolding, articulation, reflection, and elaboration of ideas (Collins et al., 1987) can be used when teaching students online.

The first three teaching strategies, modeling, coaching, and scaffolding, "are the core of cognitive apprenticeship, designed to help students acquire an integrated set of cognitive and metacognitive skills through processes of observation and of guided and supported practice" (Collins et al., 1987, p. 16).

Modeling involves demonstrating the task so students can develop a mental model, and explaining the rationales as to why it is completed in that manner. This can be translated to providing worked examples or sharing a *think-aloud protocol* in which faculty explain the requirements of an assignment, for example. In the online environment, faculty can demonstrate problem-solving strategies by asking metacognitive questions, that is, questions they would ask themselves when working through the problem (Collins et al., 1987).

Coaching is done on a one-to-one basis as the student performs the task and is a means of customizing teaching to meet individual learning needs. This may include providing hints, reminders, or feedback (Collins et al., 1987). During online discussions, for example, when a student appears to be struggling, faculty can step in and provide suggestions that link the content under discussion to prior knowledge or recent information to help the student connect the dots.

Scaffolding means providing support to complete the task without doing it for the student. Collins and colleagues (1987) describe this activity as involving "a kind of cooperative problem-solving effort by teacher and student in which the express intention is for the student to assume as much of the task on his own as possible, as soon as possible" (p. 19). *Fading* refers to the gradual elimination of scaffolding techniques as the student becomes more accomplished at completing the task and support is no longer needed. Both of these activities can be done in an online discussion. The key here is to recognize when a student is struggling and in need of faculty intervention. Asking probing questions, linking content to what the student already knows, or providing an analogy the student can relate to from past experience are all useful tools that will help faculty understand where the student is stuck, and what it might take to help move the student forward. The purpose of the next two strategies, articulation and reflection, is to hone students' observations of expert problem solving and review their own strategies. The last strategy, elaboration, involves encouraging students to identify problems and set individual learning goals.

Articulation involves explaining. By talking about the task at hand, students can test their understanding, methods of reasoning, and problem-solving strategies so that faculty can provide guidance. Faculty can promote articulation in the clinical setting by questioning the student before or after he or she performs the task, or asking the student to think aloud and explain what he or she is doing and why. This process makes student's thought processes and understanding explicit and accessible to faculty for feedback. In the online environment, a written assignment or podcast, in which students articulate thoughts about their performance, can be employed.

Reflection involves the student reviewing his or her performance after the fact and comparing it to that of the expert. This can be done verbally, modeling articulated reflection of the expert, written in a journal, or voice recorded. Assignments involving reflection are well known in nursing education, but this step is often omitted at the end of an activity. Online, this can be done in the discussions by asking students to briefly reflect on the outcome of the discussion.

The final step in the cognitive apprenticeship model, *elaboration*, pushes students to solve problems on their own as faculty's scaffolding gradually fades, giving students control over the process (Collins et al., 1987). This is possibly the most difficult step for faculty, as they must step away and allow students to wrestle with the problem, set goals, and test hypotheses (Collins, 1988).

THE TAKE-AWAY

Adults are defined as problem-centered, motivated, active learners who are goal-oriented. How we teach should match those characteristics and promote them. Regardless of what generation they belong to, most of our students are nontraditional learners who demonstrate some, if not all, of these characteristics. Their brains function similarly, according to cognitive science research, so perhaps that is what we should focus on when designing instruction and allow them to construct their own knowledge. We cannot do it for them. However, how we design our courses will make the difference. By centering small group discussions on authentic problems in a context that the learners can relate to, we can pique their interest, and coconstruction of knowledge will occur.

REFERENCES

Bargh, J. A., & Ferguson, M. J. (2000). Beyond behaviorism: On the automaticity of higher mental processes. *Psychological Bulletin, 126*(6), 925–945.

Brown, J. S., Collins, A., & Duguid, P. (1989). Situated cognition and the culture of learning. *Educational Researcher, 18*(1), 32–42.

Collins, A. (1988). Cognitive apprenticeship and instructional technology: Technical report. Office of Naval Research, Arlington, Va. Personnel and Training Research Programs Office. Report No: BBN-R-6899. Cambridge, MA: BBN Labs. Retrieved from http://files.eric.ed.gov/fulltext/ED331465.pdf

Collins, A., Brown, J. S., & Newman, S. E. (1987). *Cognitive apprenticeship: Teaching the craft of reading, writing, and mathematics* (Technical Report No. 403). Cambridge, MA: Bolt, Beranek and Newman. Retrieved from http://files.eric.ed.gov/full text/ED284181.pdf

Fang, B. (2015). How to avoid being a helicopter professor. *Faculty Focus: Higher Ed Teaching Strategies.* Madison, WI: Magna Publications. Retrieved from http://www.facultyfocus.com/articles/teachingcareers/how-to-avoid-being-a-heli copter-professor

Forrest, S. P., III, & Peterson, T. O. (2006). It's called andragogy. *Academy of Management Learning & Education, 5*(1), 113–132.

Garrison, D. R., Anderson, T., & Archer, W. (1999). Critical inquiry in a text-based environment: Computer conferencing in higher education. *The Internet and Higher Education, 2*(2–3), 87–105.

Ghefaili, A. (2003, Fall). Cognitive apprenticeship, technology, and the contextualization of learning environments. *Journal of Educational Computing, Design & Online Learning, 4,* 1–27.

Groarke, L. (2009). *An Aristotelian account of induction: Creating something from nothing.* Montreal, Quebec, Canada: McGill-Queen's University Press.

Jonassen, D. (1999). Designing constructivist learning environments. In C. M. Reigeluth (Ed.), *Instructional-design theories and models: A new paradigm of instructional theory* (pp. 215–239). Mahwah, NJ: Lawrence Erlbaum.

Knowles, M. S. (1973). Andragogy, not pedagogy. *Adult Leadership, 16*(10), 350–352.

Knowles, M. S. (1980). *The modern practice of adult education: From pedagogy to andragogy.* Chicago, IL: Follett.

Knowles, M. S., Holton, E. F., III, & Swanson, R. A. (2015). *The adult learner: The definitive classic in adult education and human resource development* (8th ed.). New York, NY: Routledge.

Lave, J., & Wenger, E. (1991). *Situated learning: Legitimate peripheral participation.* New York, NY: Cambridge University Press.

Mayer, R. E. (1999). Designing instruction for constructivist learning. In C. M. Reigeluth (Ed.), *Instructional-design theories and models: A new paradigm of instructional theory* (pp. 141–159). Mahwah, NJ: Lawrence Erlbaum.

McAuliffe, M., Hargreaves, D., Winter, A., & Chadwick, C. (2009). Does pedagogy still rule? *Australasian Journal of Engineering Education, 15*(1), 13–17.

Merriam, S. B. (2001). Andragogy and self-directed learning: Pillars of adult learning theory. *New Directions for Adult and Continuing Education, 89,* 3–13.

Nonaka, I., & Konno, N. (1998). The concept of "Ba": Building a foundation for knowledge creation. *California Management Review, 40*(3), 40–54.

Norman, G. R. (1999). The adult learner: A mythical species. *Academic Medicine, 74,* 886–889.

Reynolds, R. E., Sinatra, G. M., & Jetton, T. L. (1996). Views of knowledge acquisition and representation: A continuum from experience centered to mind centered. *Educational Psychologist, 31*(2), 93–104.

Savery, J. R., & Duffy, T. M. (1995). Problem based learning: An instructional model and its constructivist framework. *Educational Technology, 35,* 31–38.

Stetsenko, A., & Arievitch, I. (1997). Constructing and deconstructing the self: Comparing post-Vygotskian and discourse-based versions of social constructivism. *Minds, Culture, and Activity, 4*(3), 159–172.

Tudge, J., & Scrimsher, S. (2003). Lev S. Vygotsky on education: A cultural-historical, interpersonal, and individual approach to development. In B. J. Zimmerman & D. H. Schunk (Eds.), *Educational psychology: A century of contributions* (pp. 207–228). New York, NY: Routledge.

Vygotsky, L. S. (1978). *Mind in society: The development of higher psychological processes.* Cambridge, MA: Harvard University Press.

Wenger, E. (1998). *Communities of practice: Learning, meaning, and identity.* New York, NY: Cambridge University Press.

Wood, D., Bruner, J. S., & Ross, G. (1976). The role of tutoring in problem solving. *Journal of Child Psychology and Psychiatry, 17*(2), 89–100.

3

Backward Design and Elements of Course Design

Prior to teaching a course for the first time, faculty have decisions to make. These decisions include identifying learning outcomes, determining what content should be taught and how it should be organized and assessed, and choosing a textbook or other reading material. The order in which these decisions are made can have an impact on students' meeting the learning outcomes. This chapter describes the Backward Design process (Wiggins & McTighe, 2005) and how it has been reconceptualized for teaching online. This outcome-focused process is effective not only when planning assessments and teaching methods for an online course, but also for drilling down to the individual assignments.

Also included in this chapter is an explanation of workload for both students and faculty and how it impacts course design choices. The various elements of course design are explored, including authentic teaching and assessment options, and the use of quizzes as formative assessment.

APPROACHES TO COURSE DESIGN

When developing a course for the first time, several approaches to course development and design can be employed. Richards (2013) referred to these various methods as forward, central, and backward design, as they each relate to the starting point for course development. *Forward design* starts with identifying content. *Central design* focuses on the process of teaching (teaching methods). *Backward Design* begins with the learning outcomes.

In forward design, the method commonly employed in nursing, course development focuses on content. A textbook is chosen, the reading assignments are uniformly divided over the semester, teaching methods are considered, and types of assessments are identified (Richards, 2013). This method clearly focuses on teaching—what faculty will do—not on what students will learn.

Central course design begins with decisions related to what teaching methods will be employed. Although this method is not commonly used in higher education, given the growing popularity of online education where teaching methods are different from the classroom approach, knowing the mode of course delivery up front is important. Central course design may be more prevalent in K–12 classroom-based courses, where planning what the students will *do* during classes that span an hour to many hours is very important to the teacher. This method does focus on learning to some extent if the active process of coconstruction of knowledge—where students work together to help each other learn—is operationalized (Richards, 2013). However, when the focus is filling the day, the result can be what Wiggins and McTighe (2005) referred to as "hands on without being minds on" (p. 16), a very descriptive phrase that indicates one of the "twin sins" (p. 16) of instructional design. If constructivism is not the prevailing theory upon which building a course using this method is based, the danger is that activities will be planned to keep students busy without thought to the value for learning, a true definition of busywork. Even though processes or teaching methods are important to developing online courses and must be considered, they are not the best starting point for course development.

BACKWARD DESIGN PROCESS

Backward Design is an outcome-focused method for course creation or planning that is similar to purposeful task analysis (Wiggins & McTighe, 2005) and is useful at the course, curriculum, or program level. The basic premise is to teach for understanding, and that can occur only when the learning outcomes are clearly understood by faculty prior to developing any other aspect of the course. Here the authors use the term *understanding* in a way that is more inclusive than Bloom's second level of the cognitive domain. To Wiggins and McTighe, understanding means:

> to make connections and bind together our knowledge into something that makes sense of things (whereas without understanding we might see only unclear, isolated, or unhelpful facts). But the word also implies doing, not just a mental act: A performance ability lies at the heart of understanding. (p. 7)

Further discussion on what it means to understand is in order as understanding is the goal of teaching. Wiggins and McTighe (2005) have identified six "facets of understanding," which are listed in Box 3.1.

BOX 3.1
SIX FACETS OF UNDERSTANDING

- *Explanation* or *making sense of* content by telling (verbally or in writing) the how, what, where, and why of events, data, observation, and so on, and coming up with a solid explanation as to why it is supported by evidence. Another way to look at this explanation is having students *show their work.*
- *Interpretation* is the facet where the questions of *What does it mean to me?* and *So what?* are internalized and personalized. Students develop their own *story* as they wrestle with the content. This facet is where learning meets experience and results in ownership of a perspective.
- *Application* implies transfer, such as using knowledge and skills in different and perhaps new situations.
- *Perspective* requires the ability to *not* take what is known or taught at face value regardless of the source. It requires a certain amount of inquisitiveness, objectivity, and dispassionate curiosity, which allows logic to flow. It is the ability to step back and question to arrive independently at one's own view.
- *Empathy* is about appreciating diversity or what it is like to walk in another's shoes. It can be considered somewhat of a polar opposite from the facet of *perspective,* which requires distancing oneself to take an objective view. Empathy requires that the student set aside assumptions, beliefs, prejudices, pat responses, and knee-jerk reactions to understand others from their perspective. Empathy is closely related to insight, which perhaps can be thought of as the end game of being empathetic, that of gaining insight.
- *Self-knowledge* focuses on self-assessment fueled by metacognition and reflection, two constructs discussed in detail in Chapter 1.

For the practice of nursing, a balance must be struck between the facets of *perspective* and *empathy.* Benner, Sutphen, Leonard, and Day (1984/2010) label this as *boundary work* and note:

> In learning boundaries with patients, students learn not to merge with the patient's plight or pain or overidentify with the patient. They must also learn not to be too objective, too distant, but to be sufficiently open to the patient's experience to understand the patient's concerns and be of help. (p. 185)

To summarize in a few simple words without any intent to do injustice to its complex meaning, to understand is *to get it.* Educators intuitively understand this notion, yet it is difficult to define objectively and even more difficult to assess unless outcomes are clearly specified. The key, however, is to find teaching methods that promote understanding, and not simply convey the teacher's understanding, which results in memorization by the student, a common occurrence when lecture is used as the main teaching strategy (see Chapter 5 for an elaboration of this statement).

STAGES OF BACKWARD DESIGN

The Backward Design process of course design includes three sequential stages that must be aligned (Wiggins & McTighe, 2005):

1. Identify desired learning outcomes (understandings, goals, and objectives)
2. Determine evidence to demonstrate these outcomes have been met (assessments)
3. Choose learning experiences and teaching methods

Stage One

The first stage—that of determining outcomes—is more than writing behavioral objectives to indicate the learning that should occur. Fundamentally, this stage involves faculty understanding how the course being developed fits into the curriculum for the program. In other words, understanding what knowledge, skills, and attitudes students must take away from your course because content that will not be taught anywhere else must be carefully explored. This content may be *applied* in other courses, but knowing what content is unique to your course and on what level it should be taught is essential.

For example, students learn about lung function in a prerequisite anatomy and physiology course. When developing the content to accompany a clinical course, students will need to understand lung function *as it applies to* caring for a patient with chronic obstructive pulmonary disease. Thus, instead of revisiting basic lung function in detail, learning about the various methods of assessing pulmonary function would be more appropriate for a clinical course. In order for students to fully understand pulmonary function tests, they may need to revisit basic information that could be accomplished through independent study and not taught directly. So, faculty need the *big picture* of the curriculum in order to understand the contribution their course makes to the overall program. In addition, content required by the accreditation and other regulatory bodies must be considered.

The first step of identifying outcomes is to become clear on the overarching goals of learning for the course. Details on the appropriate *format* for writing goals and objectives are discussed in Chapter 4. However, to gain clarity on the goals themselves, Wiggins and McTighe (2005) recommend a few *essential* questions faculty should ask themselves. These questions are as follows: What should students know, understand, and be able to do? What content is worthy of understanding? What *enduring* understandings are desired? (p. 17).

Although these questions will point faculty to important content, keep in mind that limitations exist in that not every aspect of the topic can be taught in one course, so reasonable priorities need to be set. To further assist you in identifying important content from all possible content, Wiggins and McTighe (2005) distinguish between "worth being familiar with," "important to know," and what they term "big ideas and core tasks" (p. 71). Content that is worth being familiar with and important to know is anchored by the big ideas and core tasks. Let us take a brief detour from Stage One to explore what is meant by these concepts.

Big Ideas

As defined by Wiggins and McTighe (2005), big ideas are the

> core concepts, principles, theories, and processes that should serve as the focal point of instruction and assessment. By definition, big ideas are important and enduring. Big ideas are transferable beyond the scope of a particular module. . . . Big ideas are the building material of understandings. (pp. 338–339)

For example, diagnostic reasoning is at the core of advanced nursing practice, yet teaching the *theory* of hypothetico-deductive reasoning or pattern recognition with the goal of students subsequently being able to *apply* these theories may not yield the desired results. Diagnostic reasoning is a big idea that can be built into authentic teaching methods and assessments indirectly via the case study method. Another example of a big idea is that of using evidence to guide practice. This is a topic that may be essential content in a foundational graduate course for advanced practice nurses and a big idea in subsequent courses. Wiggins and McTighe refer to a big idea as the "linchpin" or "conceptual Velcro" (p. 66): ideas at the core of understanding that organize otherwise fragmented content and help students make sense of it.

Core Tasks

Core tasks are those skills that are essential for the role. When talking about skills in nursing, thoughts immediately migrate to clinical skills such as starting an IV or assessing heart sounds. Those are skills in the narrow sense. Wiggins and McTighe (2005) describe skills as "performance demands" (p. 78), which broaden the construct to include the complex tasks nurses do, such as reviewing patient data, assessing the patient's status, extracting the salient features, and then analyzing the results to arrive at a plan of action. Core tasks are essentially understandings-in-action.

A note of caution here. When thinking about big ideas and core tasks, one can quickly lose sight of the three steps of Backward Design, as this mental activity seems to be focused on identifying content. Keep in mind that the purpose of identifying these big ideas and core tasks is to develop a list of desired outcomes as part of the first step of the Backward Design process. The next step is to write broad goals for teaching that will become the foundation for developing learning outcomes for students, written in the form of behavioral objectives, which is discussed in Chapter 4. Suffice to say that identifying outcomes and subsequently either writing behavioral course objectives or reviewing those that were developed by the curriculum committee is the final part of Stage One.

Stage Two

Returning to the stages in the Backward Design process, the second stage of the process involves choosing the types of assessments that will determine whether the desired learning has occurred (Wiggins & McTighe, 2005). Placing this step before a decision is made on teaching methods may seem counterintuitive, but it really places the focus on assessing the learning outcomes (the objectives) instead of the minute aspects of content taught. Because the goal of teaching is for *understanding,* the facets of understanding should be revisited here as a guide as you work on Stage Two. Some of the assessments appropriate for teaching online are discussed later in this chapter under the Elements of Course Design section.

Stage Three

The third and final stage of the Backward Design process is to determine which teaching methods will promote learning at the *desired* level or the level indicated by the specific verbs that appear in the course objectives. By *learning at the appropriate level,* I am referring to the three taxonomies— cognitive, affective, and psychomotor—that describe levels of learning along a continuum. The types of assessments and teaching methods chosen must align with the level of verb in the objective. This alignment will be better understood after reading Chapter 4.

Questions suggested by Wiggins and McTighe (2005) that faculty can ask themselves in this stage are as follows:

1. What teaching methods will result in understanding?
2. What teaching materials and readings are needed to support learning for understanding?

Upon completion of these three steps, you are ready to write the objectives for the course and create the syllabus. When drilling down to the lesson level, it is helpful to repeat the steps of Backward Design to create the lessons or modules of the course to maintain your focus on learning outcomes.

Summary of Original Backward Design Process

To recap, the Backward Design process as conceived by Wiggins and McTighe (2005) is based on teaching for understanding and comprises three stages and action steps. They are summarized in Box 3.2.

BACKWARD DESIGN RECONCEPTUALIZED FOR ONLINE COURSES

The Backward Design process was originally conceived for use in classroom-based courses where summative assessment methods, or assessment *of* learning, and teaching methods were two discreet entities. However, in

---

BOX 3.2
SUMMARY OF THE ORIGINAL BACKWARD DESIGN PROCESS

1. Identify desired learning outcomes:
   a. Write goals
   b. Write or review behavioral objectives
2. Determine evidence to demonstrate meeting these outcomes:
   a. Determine types of assessments that will indicate learning has occurred (summative assessment)
   b. Determine opportunities for formative assessment
3. Choose learning experiences and teaching methods:
   a. Match teaching methods with content considering the desired performance and level of learning required
   b. Determine sequence of instruction and assessment

designing a course for the online environment, the distinction between teaching methods and assessments is blurred. In traditional classroom instruction in nursing, for example, midterm and final multiple-choice exams have been used to assess learning outcomes as summative assessments. Due to inherent difficulties, such as the potential for cheating in the online environment, in addition to the questionable value of this type of assessment to assess learning over all, the use of multiple-choice exams is changing. Frequent low-stakes quizzes are now often employed in the online environment as formative assessments and student self-assessment to promote learning from the readings and provide practice on certification exam-style questions. In addition, online group discussions provide opportunities for both formative and summative assessments. For now, it is important to begin to visualize how the indistinct line between teaching and assessment impacts online course development using the Backward Design process.

When developing an online course with the foundational underpinnings that include constructivism, social constructivism, and andragogy, all concepts discussed in Chapter 2 under the headings so named, small group discussions will most likely be the primary method of teaching, if not the teaching method of choice. Whenever student discussions are included, faculty facilitate the discussions, scaffold student learning, and provide feedback for individual students as well as on the group's overall progress toward meeting the learning outcomes. These activities, which are considered types of formative assessment, will result in reflection, potential revision of their position, and learning. Eventually, these discussions will be graded (summative assessment). Consequently, the choice of teaching methods must be considered *concurrently* with assessments. This approach compresses the second and third steps of the Backward Design process into one. The Backward Design process reconceptualized for creating online courses is summarized in Box 3.3.

The Backward Design process maintains initial focus on assessments to measure the outcomes indicated in the objectives, but also considers the

---

BOX 3.3
THE BACKWARD DESIGN PROCESS RECONCEPTUALIZED
FOR ONLINE COURSE DESIGN

1. Identify desired learning outcomes
2. Determine methods of assessment that include opportunities for formative and summative assessments as well as methods of teaching

potential for doing double duty as teaching methods. This approach to course design eliminates the need to identify additional means of assessment in the form of assignments that could result in busywork for the students.

THE ONLINE COURSE SYLLABUS

The course syllabus is an important document that guides teaching, learning, and organization of the learning management system (LMS). When developing a syllabus, West and Shoemaker (2012) recommend that faculty consider what it is like to be an online student who must juggle multiple courses, work, and family life. These students are most likely millennials who, according to Wilson and Gerber (2008), seem to struggle in courses that lack structure, but a well-thought-out syllabus can provide this needed structure. If students are to be successful, self-directed learners, we must give them enough direction from the start in order to do so.

Purpose of a Syllabus

Course syllabi serve multiple purposes. Smith (2005) identified 51 competencies required for those who plan to teach online. Some of these competencies were related to the course syllabus and helped to define its purpose, such as clearly outlining course requirements, clear explanation of what the term *participation* means, and how points will be allocated. Matejka and Kurke (1994) mentioned that a syllabus functions as a contract, means of communication, a plan, and cognitive map. In addition, a syllabus serves faculty as a planning tool to organize thoughts and schedule events (teaching and assessment).

A syllabus serves a very important function for faculty in that it demonstrates evidence of application of appropriate pedagogy (assessment strategies and teaching methods) for promotion, tenure, and accreditation. A syllabus is a permanent record of what occurred in the course and an indication to various stakeholders whether the course was appropriately designed in order to support student learning. For this reason and others, faculty should keep copies (both electronic and hard copies) of every syllabus they create. Ideally, someone at the school should be in charge of collecting and archiving all syllabi.

Because faculty spend an undue amount of time organizing a syllabus prior to teaching an online course for the first time, they are intimately familiar with the course schedule by the time the course begins. Students, on the other hand, may take a cursory look at the syllabus before classes begin and then set it aside, not fully internalizing its contents. At least that has been my experience, for multiple questions often arise 2 weeks into the course, the answers to which can be found in the syllabus. This can be frustrating for faculty, but should be kept in perspective. Strategies to avoid repeatedly having to remind students where to find information by answering multiple, individual e-mails are discussed in Chapter 12.

According to Slattery and Carlson (2005), students do rely on the syllabus in order to organize their time, especially if they are taking more than one course concurrently. Parkes and Harris (2002) provided a unique, *student-centered* perspective that is especially relevant for a constructivist paradigm.

> A learning-centered syllabus will provide information about how to plan for the tasks and experiences of the semester, how to evaluate and monitor one's performance, and how to allocate time and resources to areas in which more learning is needed. (p. 58)

This is truly how faculty hope students will use a syllabus.

From my perspective, a syllabus is a means of communication among faculty, students, and other stakeholders; a road map; and a *contract* among the students, teaching faculty, and the school. To underscore its importance as a legally binding agreement, some schools require students to sign that they have read the syllabus and had all questions addressed (Matejka & Kurke, 1994). A syllabus has also been useful to settle disputes when students have challenged grades (Parkes & Harris, 2002; Slattery & Carlson, 2005). Matejka and Kurke noted that many student frustrations and problems that arose during a course could be traced to inadequacies in the course syllabus, or policies well stated in the syllabus that were not followed once the course was underway.

Another important use of the syllabus is as a basis for equivalence when a student requests to have a course from one institution transferred to another for credit. A syllabus contains not only the course description and objectives, but also an overview of the entire course design, including reading assignments and assessments (Parkes & Harris, 2002). A quick review of a syllabus from another school will indicate if the two courses are academically equivalent. Course faculty who are the content experts are often called upon to complete this review.

Organization of an Online Syllabus

West and Shoemaker (2012) stress the need to organize the syllabus well so students can find information. The ideal situation for a school or program is to create a standardized syllabus format that faculty throughout the program or college will use. A template can be created in which certain fields can be altered by faculty to include their course-specific information, whereas those that are mandated by the school cannot be changed. When all syllabi contain the same headings, students can find information easily and appreciate the consistency.

A standardized syllabus will also partially assure that the overall look and feel is professional, but what faculty add requires careful attention. Parkes and Harris (2002) caution that: "A syllabus that is contradictory, sloppy, misleading, and incomplete models a lack of respect and of care which the students may well resent or even emulate" (p. 58). My perspective is that if we expect students' work to include proper grammar, punctuation, syntax, and American Psychological Association (APA) formatting, then what we produce should model this professional format and writing style. A hastily prepared syllabus that was copied from the previous time the course was taught requires special scrutiny to assure that all dates are correct, the textbook edition reflects the version being used, and the course description and objectives are current.

Organizing the information in a syllabus follows a logical progression. Exhibit 3.1 suggests the order and headings for a syllabus. Exhibit 3.2 depicts a Course Schedule in the syllabus that outlines how the dates and weeks are grouped in the course; educational topics, activities, and reading assignments; and the beginning and ending dates for discussions. A narrative at the top of Exhibits 3.2 and 3.3 provides additional information related to the content of the exhibit. Exhibit 3.3 demonstrates an Assessment Template in the syllabus that indicates the name of the assignments, dates they are due, the potential points for the assignment, and the actual points earned by the student. Note that midterm and final are not included in this grid. The reason for this will become evident in Chapter 8. Quizzes are, however, appropriate to help students learn course content, as formative assessments. If quizzes will be used in your course, they should be included in the Assessment Template.

EXHIBIT 3.1
Recommended Order of Information on the Syllabus

Heading	Content
Course title	Course-specific information—center course title and left justify the other headings
Course number	
Term and credit hours	
Prerequisites	

(continued)

EXHIBIT 3.1
Cognitive Case Map Example (*continued*)

Heading	Content
Faculty name(s) Contact e-mail Contact phone Skype contact	List for each faculty in this order. Indicate the lead faculty first if more than one name is listed. This person should be the go-to faculty for questions. Include preferred means to communicate with faculty.
Faculty availability	List *virtual office hours* and whether appointments are needed outside of office hours
Course description	Obtain from course catalog
Objectives	Obtain from Office of Academics
Texts • Required • Recommended	Distinguish between required and recommended texts. The listing of all texts should be in APA format with ISBN at the end of the reference.
Course schedule	List week-by-week or biweekly schedule by topic with range of dates (starting and ending) that includes reading assignments from course text and timing of discussion boards. If additional readings are required and will be linked in the LMS, list "additional readings are posted in course." *See Exhibit 3.2 for format of this section.*
Assessments	List assessments with points or percentages as they relate to the total for the course, due dates in specified time zone and types of assessments—discussions, quizzes, group projects, papers, and other assignments. Grading rubrics should be included at the end of the syllabus. *Exhibit 3.3 demonstrates recommended formatting for this section.*
Late assignments • School policy • Faculty policy	Indicate late-assignment or missed quiz/exam policies— list both the school's and yours if different
Attendance • At start of course • Continued presence	Define what students need to do to meet initial attendance requirements and to be considered as academically active throughout the course
Technical support	List contact information (e-mail and phone) and hours of availability for technical support
Policies	List institutional or program-specific policies or procedures that are required to be included in course syllabi. Most schools have a student handbook and a university policies website. Repeating information from these documents should not be done unless mandated.

APA, American Psychological Association; LMS, learning management system.

Adapted from Altman and Cashin (1992), Ko and Rossen (2010), Parkes and Harris (2002), West and Shoemaker (2012), as well as the author's experience.

EXHIBIT 3.2
Course Schedule

Following is the course schedule for the spring semester 2017. The weeks will start on Monday and end on Sunday. All discussions will start on a Monday at 8:00 a.m. and end a week from the following Friday at 11:55 p.m. Eastern Time. Posting over the weekend is optional and will be considered when grading.

Weeks	Dates	Topic/Activities	Readings
1	1/9–1/15	Introductions, orientation to course, download syllabus, begin readings	List readings from text here. Additional readings from journals are linked in LMS.
2–3	1/16–1/29	Topic (in general, not topic of discussion) Discussion 1	
4–5	1/30–2/12	Topic Discussion 2	
6–7	2/13–2/26	Topic Discussion 3	

The exhibit shows a 7-week course as an example only. The grid can be expanded to accommodate any course length.

LMS, learning management system.

EXHIBIT 3.3
Assessment Template

Following are the assessments for the course. All assessments are due on Sunday at 11:55 p.m. Eastern Time on the dates specified. See the Late-Assignment Policy in that section of the syllabus so you are aware of what to do if something occurs and your assignment will be late. I am flexible and willing to work with you *if I am made aware via e-mail before the due date and time of the assignment.* Specific criteria for the assignments and discussions can be found in the rubrics also used for grading that can be found at the end of the syllabus.

Due Date	Assignment	Potential Points	Earned Points
2/5/17	Name of assignment	10	
3/26/17	Name of assignment	10	
[a]	Discussions 1–6 (10 points each)	60	
4/23/17	Name of assignment	20	
Total		100	

[a]For dates of discussions, consult Exhibit 3.2.

Syllabus Tone

The tone of the syllabus and the language chosen are important. Slattery and Carlson (2005) point out that the tone can be "warm and friendly, formal, condescending, or confrontational" (p. 159), with a warm and friendly tone, not surprisingly, being more effective. Mager (1997) has some good advice that is useful here. He differentiates between *demand* language and *capability* language. An example of demand language is choosing words like *will, must,* or *should* when referring to what you want students to include in an assignment. The use of these words imparts a teacher-centered, formal, and potentially authoritative tone. Capability language, which also applies more to writing course objectives, is associated with the word *can*. When writing details of an assignment, consider using the words *include* or *please include*. Demand language is off-putting, and that is not the feeling you want to convey in your syllabus.

How the Online and Classroom Syllabi Differ

Although the online syllabus has many similarities with one used in a classroom-based course, a few important differences should be stressed. The main differences arise from the affordances that the online environment provides with regard to making information readily available to students via clickable links. First, links to reading assignments, such as journal articles in the library and websites of interest, that were once part of a syllabus are now added as direct links within the LMS, saving the step of opening the syllabus to find a link to the readings. Second, the faculty's philosophy of teaching, how the course fits in with other courses students have taken, and the *geography* of the course or how things are laid out in the LMS are not included in an online syllabus. I recommend faculty mention where this information can be found in a podcast that provides an introduction to the course and syllabus. To further stress these important points, include them in a bulleted list in the first announcement posted in the course.

Many LMSs have built-in software that can be used to create a flexible, interactive syllabus that is easily reworked when the course is copied for the next semester. Although this results in a syllabus that can easily be updated should changes need to be made, a permanent copy is not created unless faculty create one. In addition, students may not be able to download the syllabus in its entirety from the software, requiring that they enter the course to check the syllabus. This may not be a problem for students who access the LMS from a handheld device. I do recommend converting all documents you create in Word, including the syllabus, to PDF files, which is a more portable format. Students can readily download and read this format on their handheld devices. Not having a permanent record of a syllabus for a course can be problematic for reasons mentioned in the Purpose of a Syllabus section earlier in this chapter.

Another requirement for an online syllabus that sets it apart from that for face-to-face classes is that assignment due dates must include the time and time zone (Ko & Rossen, 2010). When students upload an assignment to the LMS, a time stamp is automatically added that occurs within the time zone of the server on which the LMS resides, not the time zone in which the student resides. As an example, suppose you and the LMS server are on Eastern Time and one of your students lives in California on Pacific Time, 3 hours behind you. He uploads an assignment at 11 p.m. Pacific Time thinking the assignment has been posted on time. However, the server stamp reflects 2 a.m. Eastern Time. From your perspective, the assignment is late and the student will, most likely, lose points. Unless the time zone for when assignments are due is specified, a well-meaning student's assignment could be considered late. As the syllabus is a legal document that may be called into action to settle a student grievance, being as specific as possible about due dates and times is recommended.

Your school may have a late-assignment policy that pertains to all students and dictates how points are deducted as well as when an assignment will no longer be accepted. This should be included in your syllabus. If you have different requirements, that information should be detailed as well.

You might be tempted to include other pieces in the syllabus that can be linked in the LMS such as how-to instructions and directions where items can be found in the LMS. How and when assignments are to be uploaded and how to use the discussion board are instructions that should be linked in the LMS and not included in the syllabus. It is useful to include an "All Weeks" section in the course where information that will be used throughout the course, and that is not week specific, can be uploaded. An area to accommodate these documents should be created if one does not exist. Documents that will be uploaded to that section in addition to the syllabus might include a podcast to review the syllabus, the link to the discussion area where students will introduce themselves, and the welcome podcast. Depending on your course design, the links to upload assignments are sometimes added to this section. A more detailed description of the organization of the LMS in terms of interface design is discussed in Chapter 12.

Rubrics are sometimes included in the syllabus, which makes sense as they are grading criteria that should be part of the contract with students. However, I find it easier to include a brief explanation of the requirements of the assignments in the syllabus and mention that a rubric will be used to grade each assignment. Also indicate where the rubric can be found in the LMS. The same name should be used for the assignment, the rubric, and the link students will click on to retrieve it in the LMS. Consistency is important.

Defining Participation

Participation in courses that meet face to face is typically loosely defined, simply because it is difficult to track and assess, depending on the number of students in the course. From the perspectives of credit-hour equivalence and student workload, participation must be clearly defined in the syllabus for online courses, as it is often a significant part of grades.

Participation in an online course involves two constructs: that of initial or first-day attendance and an ongoing presence that signifies students are active in the course. Attendance has implications for financial aid, so most institutions have a policy to ensure that all students have signed into the course initially to signify initial attendance. However, faculty are charged with monitoring student participation in academic activities that indicate their continued attendance (Electronic Code of Federal Regulations, 2016). This must be explained to students and the term *academic activities* defined. The definition of academically related activities as of August 12, 2016, according to the department of Education and Financial Student Aid, can be found in Box 3.4.

BOX 3.4
DEFINITION OF ACADEMICALLY RELATED ACTIVITIES

- Include, but are not limited to:
  - Physically attending a class where there is an opportunity for direct interaction between the instructor and students
  - Submitting an academic assignment
  - Taking an exam, an interactive tutorial, or computer-assisted instruction
  - Attending a study group that is assigned by the institution
  - Participating in an online discussion about academic matters
  - Initiating contact with a faculty member to ask a question about the academic subject studied in the course
- Do not include activities where a student may be present, but not academically engaged, such as:
  - Living in institutional housing
  - Participating in the institution's meal plan
  - Logging into an online class without active participation
  - Participating in academic counseling or advisement

Source: Electronic Code of Federal Regulations (2016).

Academic Activities and Initial Attendance

Although most of the focus from a student-aid perspective is documenting when a student ceases to attend classes, it is obviously important to determine that he or she was in class in the first place. Consequently, most schools require that after the first 7 to 10 days of a term, faculty report students who have not signed into an online class and participated in an *academically related activity* as defined in the previous section. However, most of the activities listed may not necessarily be undertaken in the first week of an online course. I recommend asking the administration to define academically related activity for that first week of class so everyone is on the same page. Note that simply logging into an online course is insufficient evidence to determine attendance. Downloading the syllabus is a reasonable inclusion in that list, in my view. Asking students to take a brief quiz regarding the functionality of the LMS, plagiarism, and the particulars included in the syllabus, for example, would be another option that would constitute initial attendance.

Academic Activities and Continued Attendance

Monitoring continued student involvement in an online course falls on faculty and can be easily forgotten once the course is in full swing. Each school must define what time frame to use. A student who is not academically active in the course for a period of time—typically 3 weeks—risks being dropped from the course. This does not happen automatically, but instead relies on faculty to inform administration of the lapse. The best approach is to contact the student via e-mail or phone to determine what the problem is before you set the course-drop process in motion. However, in order for students to participate in academically related activities, you must create them and at least one activity must occur at the interval required to meet the time frame for attendance (i.e., 3 weeks if that is the administratively determined time frame).

Implications of Attendance for Course Design

Monitoring student activity in the course can readily be done if discussion board posts are tracked. I created a discussion-tracking tool that is useful for this sort of activity *if* faculty are aware of the need to do so. This tool is discussed in Chapter 11. If discussion boards are not used in your course, another means of ensuring students' continued participation must be devised such as weekly quizzes, online journal–style posting, an assignment, or a combination of these activities. Thus, keep continued attendance in mind when choosing and timing activities in your online course.

WORKLOAD ISSUES

Course design and workload are interrelated for both students and faculty. Workload dictates course design in theory; however, in reality the relationship is less clear. Operationalizing workload hours is inconsistently done, mainly because research is lacking, and the multiple variables involved are rarely consistent among courses.

Multiple variables that can impact research on faculty workload when teaching online include class size, course design, use of technology, faculty experience teaching online, faculty knowledge regarding online pedagogy, whether the course is new or has been taught before, and if faculty are teaching the course for the first time which makes it "new" to them. Different combinations of these variables create different levels of workload, making research findings inconsistent and difficult to implement.

Faculty workload at most schools of nursing follows Boyer's model of teaching, scholarship, and service (Boyer, 1990). All of these activities take time, but few studies examine how the time commitment is broken down for each. Mandernach, Hudson, and Wise (2013) conducted a study to understand how much time faculty spent in various online teaching activities, such as grading assignments, facilitating and grading discussions, and individual interactions with students. This study involved undergraduate online courses with 20 students in each course and each instructor responsible for four, 8-week courses simultaneously. They were, however, not required to participate in committee work (service) or research. Thus, they were responsible for 80 students during the study period, a rather large number of students, in my view. The researchers found that (a) grading papers and assignments occupied 36.93% of their time weekly or 14.77 hours (3.69 hours per course), (b) facilitating discussion threads and grading discussions accounted for 22.47% of instructional time or 9.39 hours per week (2.35 hours per course), and (c) additional contact with individual students comprised 23.53% of their workweek or 9.45 hours (2.36 hours per course).

For their 40-hour workweek, over 33 hours were spent in teaching activities in four courses, 8.4 hours for each course. However, the up-front course design, syllabus creation, and setting up the LMS should be averaged over the semester and included in the total workload hours in order to have a true picture of overall faculty workload.

Because online teaching has become so prevalent in schools of nursing, faculty workload has been a topic of much debate and an issue for faculty retention (Cohen, Hickey, & Upchurch, 2009). Blackmon (2016) synthesized the literature from 2002 until 2012 to determine whether the concerns and motivations for teaching online had changed over the years. Included in her study were 24 articles, 15 of which mentioned a concern over workload and time constraints when teaching online. Although this specific theme was present in 63% of the studies, workload remained the most consistent concern in the literature during that 10-year period. Thus, concerns over faculty workload persist.

Overall, the faculty comments included in Blackmon's (2016) article reflected the inordinate amount of time spent preparing the course and teaching online, time spent reading posts and responding to students, and time away from other required faculty responsibilities. However, other aspects of the faculty's comments, listed in Box 3.5, focused on time spent in activities that reflected questionable good instructional design decisions. These concerns are revisited in Chapter 5 (see section Strategies to Offload Workload).

What these quotations represent, in my view, is a lack of understanding of online pedagogy that perhaps reflects the time period in which the study was done. Through additional educational research, we now have a better understanding of online pedagogy—what works and what does not—but much work remains to be done. All of the issues mentioned earlier when approached from a different perspective can be managed, in my view. This issue is addressed in Chapter 5 (see section Strategies to Offload Workload).

Course design and knowledge of online pedagogy are two areas that impact workload over which faculty do have control. My experience has been that online courses can be creatively designed with consideration to both student and faculty workload that will meet the learning outcomes without overtaxing either. Again, efficient strategies are discussed in Chapter 5.

BOX 3.5
FACULTY'S COMMENTS FOCUSED ON TIME SPENT
IN ONLINE TEACHING ACTIVITIES

- "With 30–40 students, to give them each individual feedback on everything they write, every week, becomes sort of daunting . . ." (Coppola, Hiltz, & Rotter, 2002 as cited in Blackmon, 2016, p. 71).
- "Faculty had to write out comments they would usually provide verbally" (Siedlaczek, 2004, as cited in Blackmon, 2016, p. 71).
- "If you're trying to write lectures or prepare PowerPoints or activities, and keep up with the dialogue, you can't do it. I learned that early enough; you can't do both. You have to really prepare your materials whether or not they are in exact final format" (Conceição, 2006, as cited in Blackmon, 2016, p. 71).
- ". . . some faculty members compared preparing to teach online courses to writing a textbook to explain the textbook" (Fish & Gill, 2009, as cited in Blackmon, 2016, p. 71).

The Credit Hour and Workload

The Carnegie Unit has been used as the basis for faculty workload, student credit earned toward a college degree, and other administrative functions since the early 1900s (Silva, White, & Toch, 2015). Originally created for K-12 education, it was based on "seat time" or the time students spent in a classroom. For higher education, a Carnegie Unit was eventually translated into a student hour (now referred to as *credit hour* or *contact hour*), which represented "an hour of lecture, of lab work, or of recitation room work, for a single pupil, with the standard college course comprising three such hours of weekly contact between students and professors over three-and-a-half-months-long semesters" (p. 9). As most college courses are 3-credit-hour courses, this translates to 3 hours per week *in class* for 15 weeks, the typical length of an academic semester. This does not include the time students are expected to spend preparing for class. Although schools have some flexibility in defining student workload, the federal guidelines for a 3-credit-hour course are:

> that the institution determine that there is an amount of student work for a credit hour that reasonably approximates not less than one hour of class and two hours of out-of-class student work per week over a semester for a semester hour or a quarter for a quarter hour. ("Program Integrity Questions," 2016, para 6)

That means that students must, on average, devote 9 hours per week to attending class and studying in preparation for class. Thus, for a 3-hour college course this equates to 135 hours over the course of a 15-week semester (Simonson, 2008).

Online courses must be academically equivalent to classroom-based courses in terms of the same student workload. Since students taking an online course do not attend class or are not in one place at the same time for the same period of time, determining workload to fill, but not overfill, the required 9 hours per week can be a challenge. The following section provides guidelines on how to accomplish this.

ELEMENTS OF COURSE DESIGN

Elements of course design that are discussed in this section include thoughts on reading assignments, textbook choice and additional readings, and the quantity of assignments beyond small group discussions. Additional course design elements are discussed in subsequent chapters and include case development (Chapter 6), discussion questions (Chapter 7), and online testing (Chapter 8). The goal in designing a course is to provide the needed educational resources to prepare students to successfully meet the learning outcomes without creating busywork. This is a fine line to walk and one for which direction and guidance is scarce. However, these are decisions you will need to make before you can finalize your syllabus.

Reading Assignments

The question of how much reading should be assigned is another academic legend, if you will, as little is written on this topic. What it has come down to is the speed at which students can read and type, the reading requirements of a typical discussion board, and the expectation of the number of hours that students should spend for a 3-credit-hour online course. The information I compiled helped me to gauge the reading assignments and number of discussions. This was greatly enhanced by the work of Barre (2016), which is published on the Rice Center for Teaching Excellence website.

The reading speed for college students has a wide range—from 200 to 400 words per minute, with the average being 300, the same for the average adult (Rayner, Schotter, Masson, Potter, & Treiman, 2016). I would imagine that many factors contributed to that wide range such as the complexity of the material, the student's inherent interest in the assigned reading, and the student's motivation to complete the reading. To put this into perspective, the average single-spaced, written page with 1-inch margins using Times New Roman 12-point font is approximately 580 words.

Understanding how many words comprise a typical discussion board will help correlate reading speed with the quantity of information students and faculty must read. At one point, I taught for a nonprofit university that required faculty to copy and paste an entire discussion board, randomly chosen by administration, into Turnitin™ software to check for the originality of students' work, that is, plagiarism. This particular course I was teaching was part of an online masters in nursing program with a nurse educator focus that had 25 students enrolled. For each discussion, students were required to post once substantively and respond to two classmates. Copying this discussion resulted in 92 pages of text (in the same format as mentioned earlier—580 words/page). If students read at a speed of 300 words per minute, it would take almost 3 hours to read all the posts. Given that students are to spend 9 hours each week for one 3-credit-hour online course, reading posts alone may take up one third of their time.

In addition to discussion posts, reading is typically assigned from textbooks and/or professional journals, which adds to the students' workload.

From a random selection of 10 journal articles, I found that the number of words per page ranged from 163 to 1,048, depending on the font size and whether the page was divided into more than one column of text. This averages to 531 words per page. Thus, the average adult reading at 300 words per minute will be able to complete an eight-page journal article in about 24 minutes. However, reading and understanding what was read are not the same. Understanding may require rereading certain passages, reflection, or engaging in self-directed metacognitive questions.

In terms of assigned reading in a textbook, Barre (2016) advised that the average page of a textbook contains about 750 words if about 25% of the page are images; obviously more words if the entire page is text. Again, depending on reading speed and the complexity of the material, a page in a textbook would take less than 3 minutes to read. A chapter consisting of 20 pages, for example, would then take about an hour for the average adult to read, more time if it were complex content.

Of interest is that the amount of reading assigned has been a topic of conversation on faculty blogs, but not of late that I could find. Alex (2008) posed the question to colleagues, stating that he thought the rule of thumb was assigning 100 pages per week for undergraduate students and 200 pages for graduate students. The replies were mixed, ranging from 66 to 250 pages per week with some respondents adding a caveat that they knew their students would not read everything they assigned.

That faculty assign reading based on the number of pages is telling to me, which is why I was happy not to find more discussion of this practice. I was enlightened by Wesley's (2016) perspective:

> The decision requires a delicate balance between the various ability levels of students in the class, the goals and outcomes of the course, the kinds of texts being analyzed, and the methods brought to that analysis. Instead of debating whether to assign more (or less), perhaps we need to focus on how to make reading matter—that is, how to make it a more meaningful exercise in our classrooms. (para. 3)

I do hope several insights come out of this conversation. First, reading should be strategically assigned with specific goals in mind of guiding and supporting learning to meet the objectives. Second, faculty should be mindful of the amount of reading they assign, knowing the average adult reading speed that translates into time on task. Also, consider that students may be taking more than one course concurrently that has required reading. Indicating in the syllabus what reading is required and what is optional or recommended is also a good practice. Keep in mind that journal articles vary widely in the number of words per page. The best way to determine the number of words per page is to copy and paste one full page into a Word document and check the word count by highlighting the text > tools on the toolbar > word count. Third, keep in mind that the amount of assigned reading is not an indicator or true measure of the rigor in your class (Wesley, 2016).

Assessments

Other considerations that must be part of course design are the number and type of assignments (assessments) to include in the course. This is a tough one. Keep in mind that small group discussions serve as teaching methods as well as means of summative assessment. Reading all the posts is time consuming for both you and your students, especially for you if you are assigning grades using a rubric.

To consider this from another perspective, online education is the original flipped classroom. If you are unfamiliar with this novel idea that Sal Khan has been promoting, it involves students reviewing lectures as homework and then going to class to work in small groups to apply what they have studied through projects, lab experiments, or working out a case study. Basically, students must come prepared to class in order to function in class. This is the order of business in an online course. Before students can post initially in the discussion—equivalent to going to class— they must prepare by completing the readings, synthesizing the content, and composing their post. We have already established that reading the posts can take up to 3 hours each week—a third of the time students should devote to the entire course. The take-away here is that few additional assignments may be necessary to promote learning and assess the objectives. Any assignment beyond doing so is busywork.

In some instances, weekly written assignments were a way for faculty to falsely assure themselves that students were studying. Because there are only so many hours in the day, these time-consuming assignments often distracted students from completing the necessary reading. As points were allotted to these written assignments, it is not difficult to determine what students attended to. This is especially important to consider given that most of our students in online nursing courses are nontraditional students who have work and family in the equation. The other disturbing outcome of weekly assignments is that the pace of completing them on time limits students' ability to learn from them. Their focus is getting from one assignment to the next.

Choosing a Textbook

Textbook choice can be time consuming and requires planning well in advance of a course. Depending upon the process at your school, it may involve requesting a desk copy through someone in administration who then contacts the publisher's local representative. In days gone by, publishers would send out desk copies without question—and often without a request. I assume cost factors have driven the change that now requires faculty to list the course and expected enrollment in the course the text will be used for before a desk copy will be sent.

Googling the name of the text can help focus your search. You can typically find the publisher's or a retail site that will allow you to peruse the first few pages of a text, which includes the table of contents. Much can be learned from that if the chapters are well named. Reviewers' comments are also helpful. I am sure it goes without saying that, depending on the topic, the text may be outdated before it is printed. However, I realize that teaching a course without a textbook may be a radical thought for some faculty. I do believe that in some cases, journal articles and reading from websites will better serve your students. The other option is to ask a publisher for permission to use a few chapters from one of their texts or create a custom text for you.

THE TAKE-AWAY

When approaching course design, backward is best. Consider outcomes first, then assessments and teaching strategies. This will focus your assessments on the desired learning outcomes articulated in the objectives and not the minutiae of what was taught. The course syllabus is an important document providing a road map for students and an indication of your understanding and application of online pedagogy. Taking time to ensure your syllabus is complete and accurate will save time later, answer questions, and calm frustrated students.

Designing your course with consideration to faculty and student workload, but keeping learning outcomes in mind, will help you choose appropriate assessments that will assess the objectives while avoiding busywork.

REFERENCES

Alex. (2008). How many pages of reading for a graduate class? [Blog message]. Retrieved from http://alex.halavais.net/question-how-much-reading-for-a-graduate-class

Altman, H. B., & Cashin, W. E. (1992). Writing a syllabus: IDEA paper No. 27. Manhattan: Kansas State University, Center for Faculty Evaluation and Development, Division of Continuing Education. Retrieved from http://files.eric.ed.gov/fulltext/ED395539.pdf

Barre, E. (2016, July). How much should we assign? Estimating out of class workload. Rice Center for Teaching Excellence. Retrieved from http://cte.rice.edu/blogarchive/2016/07/11/workload

Benner, P., Sutphen, M., Leonard, V., & Day, L. (1984/2010). *Educating nurses: A call for radical transformation.* San Francisco, CA: Jossey-Bass.

Blackmon, S. J. (2016). Teaching online, challenges and motivations: A research synthesis. *Education Matters, 4*(1), 66–83.

Boyer, E. L. (1990). *Scholarship reconsidered: Priorities of the professoriate.* Princeton, NJ: Carnegie Foundation for the Advancement of Teaching. Retrieved from http://files.eric.ed.gov/fulltext/ED326149.pdf

Cohen, M. Z., Hickey, J. V., & Upchurch, S. L. (2009). Faculty workload calculation. *Nursing Outlook, 57*(1), 50–59.

Electronic Code of Federal Regulations. (2016). *Title 34: Education. Part 668— Student assistance general provisions. Subpart B: Standards for participation in Title IV, HEA Programs, section L-7-i.* Washington, DC: U. S. Government Publishing Office. Retrieved from https://www.ifap.ed.gov/regcomps/attachments/668.pdf

Ko, S., & Rossen, S. (2010). Creating an effective online syllabus. In S. Ko & S. Rossen (Eds.), *Teaching online: A practical guide* (3rd ed., pp. 115–142). New York, NY: Routledge.

Mager, R. F. (1997). *Preparing instructional objectives: A critical tool in the development of effective instruction* (3rd ed.). Atlanta, GA: Centre for Economic Performance Press.

Mandernach, B. J., Hudson, S., & Wise, S. (2013). Where has the time gone? Faculty activities and time commitments in the online classroom. *Journal of Educators Online, 10*(2), 1–15. Retrieved from http://files.eric.ed.gov/fulltext/EJ1020180.pdf

Matejka, K., & Kurke, L. B. (1994). Designing a great syllabus. *College Teaching, 42*(3), 115–117.

Parkes, J., & Harris, M. B. (2002). The purposes of a syllabus. *College Teaching, 50*(2), 55–61.

Program Integrity Questions and Answers—Credit Hour (CH-A3). (2016). U. S. Department of Education. Retrieved August 17, 2016, from http://www2.ed.gov/policy/highered/reg/hearulemaking/2009/credit.html#credit

Rayner, K., Schotter, E. R., Masson, M. E. J., Potter, M. C., & Treiman, R. (2016). So much to read, so little time: How do we read, and can speed reading help? *Psychological Science in the Public Interest, 17*(1) 4–34.

Richards, J. C. (2013). Curriculum approaches in language teaching: Forward, central, and backward design. *RELC Journal, 44*(1) 5–33.

Silva, E., White, T., & Toch, T. (2015). *The Carnegie unit: A century-old standard in a changing educational landscape.* Stanford, CA: Carnegie Foundation for the Advancement of Teaching. Retrieved from http://files.eric.ed.gov/fulltext/ED554803.pdf

Simonson, M. (2008). Designing the "perfect" online course (Paper 82). In *Fischler College of Education: Faculty Articles.* Retrieved from http://nsuworks.nova.edu/cgi/viewcontent.cgi?article=1081&context=fse_facarticles

Slattery, J. M., & Carlson, J. F. (2005). Preparing an effective syllabus: Current best practices. *College Teaching, 4*, 159–164.

Smith, T. C. (2005, July). Fifty-one competencies for online instruction. *Journal of Educators Online, 2*(2), 1–18. Retrieved from http://www.thejeo.com/Ted%20 Smith%20Final.pdf

Wesley, C. (2016, July 13). Do you assign enough reading? Or too much? *Chronicle of Higher Education.* Retrieved from http://www.chronicle.com/article/Do-You-Assign-Enough-Reading-/237085

West, J. A., & Shoemaker, A. J. (2012). The differences in syllabi development for traditional classes compared to online courses: A review of the literature. *International Journal of Technology, Knowledge, and Society, 8*(1), 116–122.

Wiggins, G., & McTighe, J. (2005). *Understanding by design* (2nd ed.). Alexandria, VA: Association for Supervision and Curriculum Development.

Wilson, M., & Gerber, L. E. (2008). How generational theory can improve teaching: Strategies for working with the "Millennials." *Currents in Teaching and Learning, 1*(1), 29–44.

4

Writing Behavioral Objectives

Objectives have been used for decades in nursing education to set the stage for what is expected of students and to guide faculty in planning teaching and assessment. However, nursing education is evolving and the timeworn practices of how objectives were written must evolve as well. In this chapter, I provide a global view of how objectives came to be, the domains and levels involved, and offer a new view of how to write broad, measurable objectives that aligns with the call to transform nursing education (Benner, Sutphen, Leonard, & Day, 1984/2010).

THE COURSE DESCRIPTION

Most academic courses have a course description that precedes the objectives in the course syllabus. Written from the student perspective, the course description provides a broad overview of *what students will learn* from the course. It is typically content-focused and published in the school catalogue, where all courses, the credit hours, and teaching faculty are listed. Course descriptions are usually written by the program administrators, with help or review from members of the curriculum committee. Objectives for the course are written based on the course description, are often written by the curriculum committee, and focus on what students will learn from the course. Although you may not take part in writing objectives, you may be required to approve them at a faculty council meeting. To stay on point when teaching, it is imperative that you have a solid understanding of the purpose and value of course objectives, how they will guide what and how you teach, and how assessments are derived from them.

BRIEF HISTORY OF OBJECTIVES

Constructivism was first introduced in psychology circles in the late 1960s. However, for the first half of the 20th century, behaviorism was the ruling educational theory, espousing that learning was "the acquisition and strengthening of responses" (Wilson & Myers, 2000, p. 60). A change in performance or behavior was the desired outcome of instruction for the behaviorists, and little emphasis was placed on cognitive processes. It was during this time that the cognitive and affective taxonomies were written, which served to introduce more of a learner-centered, active approach to education.

Although behavioral objectives written to direct teaching and learning have had their critics, they do serve several purposes, the main one being that of communication (Mager, 1997). Objectives provide clarity for faculty in planning the teaching strategies and assessment methods for courses and offer direction for students as to what and how they should learn to be successful (Gronlund, 1995). Objectives also ensure that courses in a specific program do not overlap in content, but build upon one another to promote learning and meet programmatic outcomes.

Bloom's (1956) initial intent when developing the cognitive taxonomy was to provide a framework for writing broad objectives that described observable performance to determine whether behavior (thinking, reasoning, and doing) had changed as a result of instruction. His other purpose was to link these outcomes statements to assessment questions that would be available to all faculty who were teaching the same content—an early conceptualization of a question bank (Anderson, 2003).

So why revisit this topic? After almost 50 years, well-written objectives continue to guide teaching and learning in higher education. However, the complexities of nursing practice require a change in how objectives are written to support performance that demonstrates the *integration* of complex skills.

In this chapter, the focus is on how to write broad behavioral objectives to support learning in a constructivist, learner-centered online environment to guide teaching and learning that are in step with today's innovations in education and answer the call for radical transformation in nursing education (Benner et al., 1984/2010).

TERMINOLOGY

In spite of negative press over the decades, the revision of Bloom's original taxonomy (Krathwohl, 2002) and the introduction of other authors' conceptualizations on writing objectives (Greeno, 1976; Gronlund, 1995), Bloom's original taxonomy has prevailed. The terminology used to describe objectives has changed over the years from *educational* to *instructional,* then to *behavioral* or *performance* (Sosniak, 1994), accompanied by refinements in how they were written. Some authors distinguish among educational, instructional, and behavioral or learning objectives (Bastable & Alt, 2014). Of interest is that Bloom did not refer to his objectives as behavioral. In fact, early on he did not label them at all.

Objectives focus on the desired learning outcomes or intended behavior changes, termed *performance.* Thus, the objectives are written in behavioral terms to describe what the *student will do.* The type of assessments and the teaching strategies to use are also indicated by the domain and level of verb chosen for the objective, but even so, they are not focused on what the teacher will do (Bloom, 1956; Gronlund, 1995). This is an important distinction. As objectives are written in behavioral terms that specify desired changes in behavior or performance in terms of thinking, feeling, and doing that will occur as the result of instruction, the term *behavioral objectives* has been used throughout this chapter.

UNDERSTANDING A TAXONOMY

Writing objectives in the appropriate format is challenging, in part, because of the lack of a clear understanding of what the term *taxonomy* means. A taxonomy is a hierarchical classification system that is structured from simple to complex and general to abstract (Gronlund, 1995; Krathwohl, 2002). In other words, the hierarchical structure requires that preliminary levels be mastered before learning at higher levels can occur. For example, in the cognitive domain, the levels are knowledge, comprehension, application, synthesis, analysis, and evaluation indicating increasingly complex skills. In order to apply a concept, one must have knowledge of it and understand it (Gronlund, 1995).

This requirement does not, however, dictate that knowledge must be taught directly, requiring students to memorize isolated facts so they can be applied later. Keep in mind that most students taking an online nursing course are RNs returning to school who have all completed one of the basic nursing programs whose content is dictated by the accreditation process and therefore is quite homogeneous. Foundational facts and concepts can be taught indirectly within an authentic constructivist context through case studies, for example. This type of teaching method requires students to recall what they already know about the topic, identify where their understanding ends, and learn from there. This topic is discussed in greater detail in Chapters 6 through 8. At this juncture, it is important to understand what the term taxonomy means in educational contexts and to understand its inherent hierarchal nature.

Bloom's taxonomies include a numbering convention typical of a taxonomy. The domains or classes, as Bloom (1956) called them, are numbered with whole numbers and two decimal points. Subclasses are identified by changes in the first or second decimal. Box 4.1 provides an example of the classes of the cognitive domain showing expanded subclasses of the *comprehension* level. Consequently, objectives and subobjectives can be numbered as well, although this is rarely done. This numbering is mentioned here to give the reader the full picture of the organization of the taxonomy and an understanding of the numbering convention should it be encountered at some point.

Bloom's (1956) original taxonomy focused on the cognitive domain with that of the affective taxonomy following about 10 years later (Krathwohl, Bloom, & Masia, 1964). Bloom did not develop a taxonomy for the psychomotor domain, mainly because he felt that the learning outcomes of the core courses at the University of Chicago, where he was teaching at the time, did not lend themselves to this type of learning. He did, however, recognize that psychomotor learning required a different set of learning outcomes. Several versions of a taxonomy for the psychomotor domain were later developed (Dave, 1970; Harrow, 1972; Simpson, 1966), with Simpson's work gaining the most widespread use.

To Bloom and his colleagues (Krathwohl et al., 1964), the purpose of learning was to change students' behavior in terms of their ability to "act, think, and feel" (Bloom, 1956, p. 12). The purpose of the taxonomies was to classify levels of learning in three domains (cognitive, psychomotor, and

---

BOX 4.1
NUMBERING SYSTEM FOR A TAXONOMY

1.00 Knowledge
2.00 Comprehension
   2.10 Translation
   2.20 Interpretation
   2.30 Extrapolation
3.00 Application
4.00 Analysis
5.00 Synthesis
6.00 Evaluation

affective) for the purpose of communication on several levels (Anderson, 2003). The names and brief definitions of these domains are:

1. Cognitive: thinking
2. Psychomotor: acting or doing
3. Affective: emotions, values, and attitudes

Objectives written in each of these domains served to provide a common language that formed the basis for designing assessments and instruction (Gronlund, 1995), as well as communicating expectations of learning and assessment to students, which Felder and Brent (1997) dubbed "an advance warning system" (p. 179).

THE COGNITIVE DOMAIN

The Lower Levels of the Cognitive Domain

The cognitive domain "includes those objectives that deal with recall or recognition of knowledge and the development of intellectual abilities and skills" (Bloom, 1956, p. 7). This domain consists of six levels that are arranged in a hierarchy from concrete to abstract. The levels are knowledge, comprehension, application, analysis, synthesis, and evaluation, in that order. Each higher level subsumes mastery of the lower levels. The first three levels, considered to be lower cognitive functions, as described in Bloom's (1956) original taxonomy, are listed in Box 4.2.

Transfer of Learning and the Cognitive Domain

At this juncture, it is important to revisit the concept of transfer and understand how it fits into the levels of the taxonomy, as well as reiterate the structure of a taxonomy. Remember that a taxonomy is a hierarchy from concrete to abstract that requires mastery of the lower levels prior to moving on to higher learning outcomes. In other words, one cannot apply a concept, principle, and so forth without first knowing about it (knowledge level) and understanding (comprehension level) how to use it. Mastery of the comprehension level, as first described by Bloom (1956), meant that the student could use knowledge gained in the same or similar situation in which it was taught, indicating *understanding*. In this instance, Bloom was referring to *near transfer* (Merriam & Leahy, 2005). *Far transfer* occurs at the application level, when students apply what was learned to new and novel situations. The concept of transfer has been discussed in detail in Chapter 1.

BOX 4.2
LOWER LEVELS OF BLOOM'S ORIGINAL COGNITIVE DOMAIN

1. *Knowledge*—Bloom (1956) defined knowledge as "those behaviors and test situations which emphasize the remembering, either by recognition or recall, of ideas, material, or phenomena" (p. 62).
2. *Comprehension*—Bloom (1965) defined comprehension as "those objectives, behaviors, or responses which represent an understanding of the literal message contained in a communication" (p. 89). The act of understanding involves three steps: translation, interpretation, and extrapolation. *Translation* is the first step in meaning-making as learners translate what they have learned into their own words. *Interpretation* involves "dealing with a communication as a configuration of ideas whose comprehension may require a reordering of the ideas into a new configuration in the mind of the individual" (p. 90). From this reconfiguration may arise new "inferences, generalizations, or summarizations" (p. 90) in order to make sense to the individual. *Extrapolation* is demonstrated when the individual makes "inferences in relation to implications, consequences, corollaries, and effects which are in accordance with the conditions described in the communication" (p. 90). This signifies understanding.
3. *Application*—The application level involves using acquired knowledge and understanding in new and novel situations. This is the definition of far transfer (Chapter 1), which is the goal of education (Anderson & Sosniak, 1994; Mayer, 1998; Merriam & Leahy, 2005). When given a new problem to solve, this level stipulates the ability to "apply the appropriate abstraction without having to be prompted as to which abstraction is correct or without having to be shown how to use it in that situation" (p. 120).

From a slightly different perspective, consider his conceptualization of near transfer (comprehension level) and far transfer (application level) in view of the assumptions of adult learning theory. One of these assumptions is that adults are intrinsically motivated to learn in preparation for new roles and responsibilities, which is, in turn, related to their need for immediate application of what was learned (Forrest & Peterson, 2006). Students taking online courses are most likely RNs who are continuing their education because they have a specific goal in mind. If that involves a role change (nurse practitioner, educator, researcher, or administrator), they are most likely familiar with the role functions and the additional knowledge they must acquire to function in that role. And they are motivated to acquire it. Most students are self-directed in their approach and do not expect to be spoon-fed. Teaching content within context will engage students, allow them to think like a nurse practitioner, administrator, researcher, or educator, and help them transfer what they are learning to their new role in order to function in the real world (Benner et al., 1984/2010; Tanner, 2006). This approach will avoid the need for faculty to teach everything students need to learn for the role they aspire to. Transferring what is learned to similar or new situations will naturally occur if the context in which learning occurs is similar to real life (authentic) and has meaning to the learner in that he or she can readily see its application.

In addition, adult students bring a wealth of experience to the learning environment, and no two students have the same experiences. The same can be said for acquired knowledge, even though the knowledge transmitted in basic nursing programs is standardized. As what is learned depends on what is already known (Lalley, & Gentile, 2009; Reynolds, Sinatra, & Jetton, 1996) and that is based on the combination of knowledge and experience, the assumption can be made that because students' baseline knowledge differs, they will learn at different levels and transfer new knowledge in unique ways.

The Higher Levels of the Cognitive Domain

Returning to the definitions of levels in the cognitive domain in the original taxonomy, Bloom (1956) defined *analysis, synthesis,* and *evaluation* as requiring *higher cognitive skill* and they subsequently became known as *higher order* levels of the taxonomy. Controversy exists as to whether the application level should be included in that group (Marken & Morrison, 2013). As application requires the ability to transfer and the goal of education is for students to transfer what they have learned to their future role (Anderson & Sosniak, 1994; Mayer, 1998), I believe that the application level should be the lowest level at which objectives should be written to achieve desired learning outcomes. When students apply what they know, they combine knowledge and skill, and subsequently use it creatively through transfer. This approach is consistent with the goals of transforming nursing education (Benner et al., 1984/2010) by "integrating all three professional apprenticeships, the knowledge base, skilled know-how, and clinical reasoning and ethical comportment, in all teaching and learning settings" (p. 80). Consequently, I believe this level should be included in the higher order group, considering the complex skill of transfer required for application.

The previously listed higher order levels of the cognitive domain include analysis, synthesis, and evaluation. Their definitions appear in Box 4.3. Based on these definitions, it is apparent how each level builds upon the previous level to arrive at what Bloom has termed "intellectual abilities and skills" (Benner et al., 1984/2010, p. 38) and Wiggins and McTighe (2005) refer

---

BOX 4.3
HIGHER ORDER LEVELS OF THE COGNITIVE DOMAIN

1. *Analysis* "emphasizes the breakdown of the material into its constituent parts and detection of the relationships of the parts and of the way they are organized" (Bloom, 1956, p. 194).
2. *Synthesis* is defined as "the putting together of elements and parts so as to form a whole" (Bloom, 1956, p. 162). Synthesis often combines knowledge and experience to create something new. Mastery of this level requires a certain level of creativity.
3. *Evaluation* is defined as "the making of judgments about the value, for some purpose, of ideas, works, solutions, methods, materials, etc. It involves the use of criteria as well as standards for appraising the extent to which particulars are accurate, effective, economical, or satisfying" (Bloom, 1965, p. 185).

---

to as "understanding," a much broader conceptualization than the second level in Bloom's taxonomy.

THE PSYCHOMOTOR DOMAIN

The psychomotor domain is the skills domain in the narrow sense of the word, in that this domain provides a means of identifying outcomes that involve fine, manual, and gross motor movements (Reilly & Oermann, 1985). Fine motor movement involves precise movement, whereas gross motor activity has to do with large muscles or movement using the entire body. The concept of manual movement is heard about less often, yet is meaningful for nursing, and is defined as "manipulative tasks that are repetitive and often involve 'eye–arm' action (e.g., physical assessment or suctioning)" (Reilly & Oermann, as cited in Oermann, 1990, p. 202). Although the desired outcomes of these objectives and therefore assessment of these objectives focus on muscle movement, cognitive and affective activities are also involved with psychomotor activities, more so when a new skill is being learned (Oermann, 1990).

The accompanying cognitive and affective activity required to learn a skill differs from that of performing the skill, a distinction that should be kept in mind when teaching. Faculty often question students as to why they are doing something while they are performing. This interrupts the motor portion of skill performance, switching the student to the cognitive brain function to respond to the question. The skill performance of *doing* is interrupted by the cognitive activities of *remembering* and *recalling*, causing both performances to suffer (Bastable & Alt, 2014).

Keep in mind that when writing an objective in the psychomotor domain, the desired outcome must focus on fine, manual, or gross motor movements and not the cognitive activity required to learn the skill. Multiple-choice questions (MCQs) can be developed to assess the knowledge behind the skill to differentiate the students' understanding of the *why* that supports performance from rote memorization of the order or sequence of necessary steps. Transfer of learning can occur only if the *knowing that*, or the knowledge behind the skill, is associated with *knowing how*, or the performance of the skill. For example, when teaching sterile technique for Foley catheter insertion, students must learn the theory of asepsis, which is then applied during performance of the skill. When teaching sterile dressing change, faculty should not need to repeat the theory of asepsis. Students should be able to transfer that understanding and accurately apply it to a sterile dressing change, a new and novel situation.

Levels of the Psychomotor Domain

Simpson (1966) identified seven levels in the psychomotor domain that demonstrate increasing fluidity and automaticity of skill performance, accomplished by repeated practice of the skill (Oermann, 1990). The same numbering convention used in the cognitive domain can be applied to this domain. The seven levels are shown in Box 4.4.

BOX 4.4
LEVELS OF THE PSYCHOMOTOR DOMAIN

- *Perception:* The first level involves becoming aware of the need to act through choosing the appropriate action. This first level includes three processes:
  - Becoming aware via one of the senses (auditory, visual, tactile, taste, smell, or kinesthetic) that action is required
  - Determining (from deciding to intuitive knowing depending upon experience) which cues to respond to
  - Recognizing and selecting the appropriate task

  These activities are really *cognitive.* Key concepts are cue recognition and choice of action.

- *Set:* This level involves the mental, physical, and emotional readiness to perform an action. *Mental readiness* refers to the recognition and

---

(continued)

BOX 4.4
LEVELS OF THE PSYCHOMOTOR DOMAIN (*continued*)

understanding of the task to be performed. *Physical readiness* requires focusing the necessary senses on the act to be performed, whereas emotional readiness includes having a favorable attitude and willingness to perform. This level includes cognitive and affective activities. The key concept is readiness to perform.

- *Guided response:* This level reflects performing under the guidance of a more knowledgeable individual, such as an instructor. This level has two subcategories:
  - *Observation* of faculty's performance with subsequent imitation by the learner (return demonstration) and/or observance and adoption of faculty's behavior by the student.
  - *Trial and error* plays a role in this level, which signifies the beginning of actual motor performance. Time for trial and error should be provided, as it is an important learning strategy when guided by faculty and the underlying theory of the task. Feedback, both intrinsic (student's ongoing self-evaluation) and extrinsic (augmented by faculty), is important at this level. The key concept is guided (*not independent*) performance that occurs in the process of learning.
- *Mechanism:* Confidence in and habituation of the performance distinguish this level from others. The learner has reached a certain level of comfort performing the skill and has developed a set pattern that can be relied on for future performance. Key concepts include confidence, habituation, and patterning.
- *Complex overt response:* This level is characterized by resolution of uncertainty about performance, which is now completed smoothly, efficiently, and automatically. The skill level can be considered high when this level has been reached. Key words that define performance are *smooth* and *automatic*.
- *Adaption:* This level reflects students' ability to adapt their performance to the unique characteristics of the setting and situation, which for nursing might include the physical environment and individual patient needs. Key concepts are adaptation of performance and responding to cues.
- *Origination:* This level reflects students' ability to create new patterns of performance, adhering to the underlying concepts and theories that guide performance. At this level, new approaches are taken to solve a problem and/or effective shortcuts are taken. Key concepts are new patterns of performance and creativity.

Harrow (1972), somewhat critical of this model, pointed out that behavioral changes in the first two levels, *perception* and *set,* are not readily apparent or visible to faculty, and therefore cannot be assessed directly through observation of the performance. In addition, these two levels do not include any motor activity. The first level (perception) indicates cognitive behavior, as one perceives the need to act. The second level (set) reflects cognitive and affective behavior, as one prepares to act on mental, physical, and emotional levels.

The take-away is that objectives should not be written for the first two levels as they do not indicate psychomotor behavior, and they would be very difficult to assess other than by self-report, which is really a *cognitive* activity. Faculty can assume these first two levels have been met if the student is observed performing at a higher level—that of *guided response* or above. For example, if the student is observed correctly performing the appropriate procedure, the *assumption* can be made that both the perception (identifying the need to act) and set (choosing the correct performance) levels have been mastered. Thus, if an objective is written for the psychomotor domain, the lowest level of performance that can be observed is the guided response level. The first two levels of the domain can be assessed using MCQs or by questioning the student before or after the student performs the skill.

THE AFFECTIVE DOMAIN

Krathwohl et al. (1964) developed a taxonomy of the affective domain as a means of stating learning outcomes related to "a feeling tone, an emotion, or a degree of acceptance or rejection . . . interests, attitudes, appreciations, values, and emotional sets or biases" (p. 7). The organizing concept for this hierarchy is the concept of *internalization,* which ranges from attending to an emotion, feeling, value, and so forth to becoming a part of one's character or assimilated into the self. Although the affective domain is very important for nursing, this type of objective is a challenge to write and difficult to assess, mainly because the behavioral changes that occur as a result of meeting these objectives are generally internal changes and are not observable (Martin & Reigeluth, 1999).

Although the cognitive and affective taxonomies were written as two separate hierarchies out of necessity, thinking and feeling are closely related in the human brain (Sylvester, 1995; Zul, 2002). For example, learning about a topic in greater depth will often result in students developing an attitude, value, or interest in that content. This is knowledge and understanding (cognitive activities) influencing beliefs or values (affective activities). Conversely, a young man's belief that men will not be as successful in nursing as females because exhibiting caring behavior is not manly may prevent him from entering the profession. This is an example of a belief influencing cognition.

Keep in mind that both the cognitive and affective taxonomies were written in the 1950s and 1960s before science understood how the brain learns. Research in this area within the past 25 years has brought new insights into the relationship of the *thinking brain* to the *feeling brain*. According to Sylvester (1995) and Zul (2002), emotions are involved with the individual attending to one stimulus over another in today's stimuli-laden environment, thus driving what is learned and remembered. This interrelationship is important to remember when planning learning activities.

Levels of the Affective Domain

The affective domain consists of five levels (Krathwohl et al., 1964). As in the other domains, each level can be numbered in a taxonomic fashion (1.00, 2.00, etc.). Descriptions of the five levels are listed in Box 4.5. Krathwohl et al. (1964) contended that reaching the final level is not the goal of higher education. Thus, faculty should avoid writing objectives to that level.

Although cognitive, psychomotor, and affective mental activities do not occur in isolation, but are in effect interrelated, when writing objectives it is necessary to first gain clarity on the desired learning outcome before choosing the domain and level for an objective. Also, when writing objectives it is important to keep in mind that:

- All objectives must be assessed
- From the verb chosen, objectives should indicate the domain and level of learning desired
- Objectives must contain only one learning outcome, thus one verb
- Verbs must be measurable

RECOMMENDED VERBS

When choosing a verb from the various levels of the three domains, it is best to focus first on the intended learning outcome to indicate the domain or the type of learning required. Ask yourself, does the intended outcome involve primarily thinking (cognitive); muscle movement (psychomotor); or feelings, values, or attitudes (affective)? Then consider the level of learning desired and choose the appropriate verb from that level. Keep in mind that the objective, thus the verb chosen, must reflect a performance, or

---

BOX 4.5
LEVELS OF THE AFFECTIVE DOMAIN

- *Receiving:* This first level is about the learner being "sensitized to the existence of certain phenomena and stimuli . . . that is . . . willing to receive or attend to them" (p. 98). Three levels of *attending to* on a continuum also indicate key words. These three sublevels are awareness (conscious), willingness to receive (or attend to without judgment), and controlled or selected attention by the learner (focusing on).
- *Responding:* In this level, the learner goes beyond being aware of a phenomenon and shows interest in it, reluctantly at first, but with increasing willingness. Three sublevels indicating keywords are acquiescence in responding (obedience or compliance), willingness to respond, and satisfaction in response.
- *Valuing:* This level indicates the learner's assignment of worth to a phenomenon, and the learner's behavior demonstrates increasing internalization as he or she begins to accept, demonstrate preference for by seeking out, and commit to the value. Others' perception is that the individual holds a specific value, which has become a belief. Three levels indicating key words are acceptance of a value, preference for a value (seeks it out), and commitment indicating conviction and a high degree of certainty.
- *Organization:* This level results in the development of a value system through "organization of values into a system, determination of interrelationships among them, and the establishment of the dominant and persistent ones" (p. 154). The two levels indicating key words are conceptualization of a value through abstraction and determining how it relates to other values held and organization of a value system.
- *Characterization* by a value or value complex: At this level, the individual has developed a worldview, is comfortable with it, and lives by it. Two levels indicating key words are generalized set or an attitude cluster that predisposes individuals to act in a specific way that is most likely unconscious and characterization indicating complete internalization of values.

Source: Krathwohl et al. (1964).

---

something the student will *do* or *demonstrate* (Mager, 1997). Exhibits 4.1 to 4.3 list the recommended verbs in the various domains that were compiled by a sort of Delphi technique based on the early work of the original writers or interpreters of the various taxonomies (Bastable & Alt, 2014; Bloom, 1956; Gronlund, 1995; Krathwohl et al., 1964; Oermann & Gaberson, 2014) and my extensive experience writing objectives. Exhibit 4.1 lists recommended verbs

EXHIBIT 4.1
Recommended Cognitive-Domain Verbs

Level	Description	Recommended Verbs
Knowledge	The emphasis in this level is on remembering or recalling information	Define, identify, label, list, name, recall, state
Comprehension	Behaviors requiring understanding of material	Describe, differentiate, explain, generalize, give examples of, interpret, recognize, select, summarize, write
Application	Using knowledge and understandings in a new or novel way	Demonstrate, illustrate, implement, modify, operate, relate, revise, solve, use
Analysis	Breaking material down into its constituent parts, identifying relationships between the parts, and understanding how they are organized	Analyze, classify, compare, contrast, detect, diagram, discriminate, distinguish, map
Synthesis	Combining parts into a unified whole, creating a new product or process	Categorize, combine, compile, compose, construct, correlate, create, derive, design, devise, generate, integrate, produce, reconstruct, reorganize, restructure, summarize
Evaluation	Making judgments about the value of something using criteria and/or standards	Appraise, assess, conclude, criticize, defend, extrapolate, judge, justify

Adapted from Bastable and Alt (2014), Bloom (1956), Gronlund (1995), Krathwohl et al. (1964), Oermann and Gaberson (2014), and the author's extensive experience writing objectives.

from the cognitive domain. Exhibit 4.2 lists the recommended verbs from the psychomotor domain. Exhibit 4.3 lists the recommended verbs from the affective domain.

PROBLEMATIC VERBS

The key to writing meaningful objectives is in choosing a measurable verb, as many verbs seem measurable, but are not. Verbs that must be followed by descriptors to understand what is to be learned should be a tip-off that measurability of the verb is in question, such as *develop a plan* or *understand the relationship*. In these examples, the verb does not indicate how content should be taught (at what level), the level of performance required, or the

EXHIBIT 4.2
Recommended Psychomotor-Domain Verbs

Level	Definition	Recommended Verbs
Perception	Becoming aware of the need for action, attending to the appropriate cue to act upon, and determining the type of action needed	Not assessable within the framework of the psychomotor domain. *These activities are cognitive, thus no verbs are recommended.*
Set	This level involves the mental, physical, and emotional readiness to perform an action	Not assessable within the framework of the psychomotor domain. *These activities are cognitive and affective, thus no verbs are recommended.*
Guided response	Performing under the guidance of an instructor	Illustrates, imitates, performs with guidance, tries, discovers, practices, uses trial and error
Mechanism	Performance relies on developed pattern of responses (mechanical) due to increasing comfort with the process	Accurately demonstrates or performs, carries out, follows steps or procedures, maintains
Complex overt response	Smooth, automatic efficient performance	Demonstrates with confidence, efficiently completes, performs without hesitation, skillfully demonstrates, smoothly and efficiently performs
Adaption	Ability to adapt performance to various circumstances	Adapts, alters, changes, converts, corrects, rearranges, reorganizes, replaces, revises, substitutes, switches
Origination	New patterns of performance are created while adhering to the underlying concepts and theories that guide performance	Creates new patterns or procedures, devises shortcuts

Adapted from Bastable and Alt (2014); Krathwohl et al. (1964); Oermann and Gaberson (2014); Simpson (1966); and the author's extensive experience writing objectives.

type of assessment indicated to meet the objective. Thus, the verb does not indicate the level of complexity of *doing* that is required by students. In the first example, what can be assessed is the deliverable only, *a plan*. However, the verb does not indicate what it is about the student's performance related to the plan that should be assessed. The second example requires a descriptor in the form of a prepositional phrase to understand more about the *relationship,* such as *between X and Y.* Questions to ask to determine whether the verb is measurable include:

1. Does the verb in this objective indicate both performance and a level of performance?
2. Will the verb in this objective help develop assessments and teaching strategies?
3. Will the verb in this objective inform students what they need to do to meet the objective?

EXHIBIT 4.3
Recommended Affective-Domain Verbs

Level	Description	Recommended Verbs
Receiving	Becoming sensitive to a stimuli through awareness, being receptive without judgment, and selectively focusing on specific stimuli.	Writing an objective at a higher level of the domain will better assess this level. Assessing after the fact, by asking the student to recall his or her feelings or attitudes, is a cognitive activity, not affective. *No verbs are recommended for that reason.*
Responding	Demonstrates increasing interest in the stimuli initially obediently, becoming more willing until satisfaction with response is reached.	Like the first level, writing an objective at a higher level of the domain will better assess this level. Potential verbs for this level are—acts willingly, assists, is willing to, participates
Valuing	Increasing internalization through acceptance, preference for, and commitment to a value until it has become a belief.	Appreciates, desires to attain, prefers, seeks out, assumes responsibility for, actively participates in, commits to, values
Organization	Development of values into a system through conceptualization of a value through its relationship to other values and organization of a value system.	Conceptualizes the value of, defends, derives ideas, develops a rationale, forms judgments, forms judgments as to or related to, judges, weighs alternatives
Characterization by a value or value complex	Development of a worldview, is comfortable with it, and lives by it.	Obtaining this level requires life experience over time and is not assessable in a meaningful way based on learning in one course. *No verbs are recommended here as this level cannot be assessed based on one course.*

Adapted from Bastable and Alt (2014), Krathwohl et al. (1964), Oermann and Gaberson (2014).

EXHIBIT 4.4
Problematic Verbs

Verb	Potential Issue
Discuss	This is really an activity or process and does not indicate a level of performance.
Know, understand, comprehend	These verbs are difficult to assess and may lack interrater reliability.
Apply	This can be used appropriately if what follows the verb indicates performance. For example, "apply best evidence" does not communicate the desired performance. This is better used as a descriptive phrase, such as—"determine a plan of treatment by applying best evidence." Many application verbs can be used incorrectly in the same type of instance.
Develop	The verb itself indicates a process, not a performance, and does not describe "doing." The "what" of "what is to be developed" is what describes performance, making the objective difficult to assess.

Adapted from Bastable and Alt (2014), Bloom (1956), Gronlund (1995), Krathwohl et al. (1964), Mager (1997), Oermann and Gaberson (2014), and the author's extensive experience writing objectives.

If the answer to these questions is "no," then problems exist with the verb and/or the way the objective was structured. Exhibit 4.4 lists problematic verbs with an explanation as to why they are so, again this list is compiled from multiple authors and those with various interpretations of appropriate verbs (Bastable & Alt, 2014; Bloom, 1956; Gronlund, 1995; Krathwohl et al., 1964; Oermann & Gaberson, 2014) as well as my experience. These verbs should be avoided when writing objectives.

STRUCTURE OF AN OBJECTIVE

Component Parts

Mager's (1997) seminal work on the format for writing objectives remains useful today, especially when first learning how to write broad measurable objectives. He maintained that objectives should comprise three parts: *performance, condition,* and *criterion.*

The performance component indicates, "what someone would be doing when demonstrating mastery of the objective" (Mager, 1997, p. 52). Here, it is important to focus on:

- What the student will be *doing* or *producing*
- A specific domain (cognitive, psychomotor, or affective)
- The level within that domain (knowledge, comprehension, application, etc.) of learning required
- The verb that will demonstrate the performance when assessed

The second part of an objective is more standardized in higher education than in workplace training and addresses the condition, or the circumstances that are associated with the performance (Mager, 1997). An example related to an objective for a health assessment course might be: *Using a reflex hammer, the student will demonstrate the correct technique when eliciting deep tendon reflexes.* Here, the condition is "using a reflex hammer."

Mager's (1997) objectives written for trainings were often quite specific. He believed that "you write as many objectives as you need to describe *all* instructional results you think are important to accomplish" (p. 49). Having too many objectives can tax students' cognitive load (Chapter 1) and does not capture the type of performance required of complex nursing roles. In higher education, this specificity is observed in subobjectives written at the weekly content or biweekly module level. This practice, however, is one I do not recommend, as there are better alternatives in the online environment, which are discussed in Chapter 12.

In higher education when broad performance encompassing multiple skills is desired, the condition is often written: *At the end of the course, the student will be able to. . . .* This phrase is located at the top of the list of objectives to avoid repeating the condition at the start of each objective. A broad objective that would include the skill of using a reflex hammer as well as a stethoscope, tuning fork, ophthalmoscope, and other tools might be: *At the end of the course, the student will be able to demonstrate coordinated and skillful use of diagnostic tools, such as a stethoscope, tuning fork, reflex hammer, ophthalmoscope, and otoscope, during a comprehensive physical examination.* Listing the tools here leaves little room for misunderstanding, important to keep in mind when one of the purposes of objectives is communication between students and faculty. Being specific is a practice students will appreciate when it comes time for summative assessment.

A few words are in order on the debate that exists about the wording of the condition. Which wording seems more supportive of students?: (a) *at the end of the course the student will . . .* or (b) *at the end of the course the student will be able to. . . .* Mager (1997) differentiates between *demand* language, as reflected in example (a), *the student will,* compared to *capability* language noted in example (b), *the student will be able to* (p. 78). Gronlund's (1995) view is that objectives should be written with an economy of words, and he recommends using the verb *can,* another example of capability language. Writing the condition using *at the end of this course the student can . . .* is another way to express capability language. To me, capability language is more in line with what should be conveyed to students, which is the confidence the instructor has that as a result of instruction at the end of the course, they will be able to perform.

The third part of an objective is the criterion that conveys to students how well they must perform to meet the objective. This can be accomplished by adding words such as *accurate*, or a percentage such as *80% of the time*. Returning to the previous example: *At the end of the course, the student will be able to demonstrate coordinated and skillful use of diagnostic tools, such as a stethoscope, tuning fork, reflex hammer, ophthalmoscope, and otoscope, during a comprehensive physical examination,* words indicating the criteria are *coordinated* and *skillful*. Although these words may leave room for different interpretations among faculty grading the same performance, the analytic rubric used for grading can specify what is required to gain full points.

A note of caution is in order. Avoid setting *100% of the time* as the criterion, as this is often an unrealistic goal for two reasons. Based on Benner's (1984/2001) work on the novice-to-expert continuum, an expert would most likely achieve this benchmark. However, graduate students are, at the most, competent at graduation. The second reason is that unless performance is assessed more than once for that objective, which may not be possible, 100 percent of the time or referring to every time does not make much sense. The criterion may be difficult to include in some objectives, so forcing it to *comply* with the preferred format is not wise. Omit the criterion if it does not add meaning and clarity to the objective.

WRITING BEHAVIORAL OBJECTIVES

Goals and Objectives: What's the Difference?

In their landmark treatise, Benner et al. (1984/2010) called for a "more effective integration of the three professional nursing apprenticeships" (p. 82), which are "to learn nursing knowledge and science, a practical apprenticeship to learn skilled know-how and clinical reasoning, and an apprenticeship of ethical comportment and formation" (p. 25). The authors challenged nursing educators to teach with *integration* of clinical and classroom content, essentially to teach within context, so that students can associate domain knowledge, *knowing that,* with skill-based knowledge, *knowing how,* in order to prepare students for the complex nature of nursing practice.

The authors urge nursing educators to "shift from a focus on covering decontextualized knowledge to an emphasis on teaching for a sense of salience, situated cognition, and action in particular situations" (p. 82). This call to action will require a transformation of our thoughts on both teaching and learning, stepping away from a role of *conveyor of knowledge* to that of a catalyst for learning. This shift requires a hard look at how we think about goals and objectives.

To achieve an endpoint of integrated knowledge and skills, I propose a reconceptualization of how objectives are written. Some authors have made a distinction between goals and objectives. Goals have been considered as the desired outcome of instruction in the long term (Bastable & Alt, 2014) and the precursors of objectives (Mager, 1997), whereas objectives have been defined as indicating "a specific, single, unidimensional behavior" (Bastable & Alt, 2014, p. 386) achievable in the short term. Objectives related to goals must be met before that goal can be achieved. Thus, writing specific objectives often resulted in a lengthy list for a course, but then subobjectives were written for each week or module. When referring to the changes in terminology associated with writing objectives, Sosniak (1994) lamented:

> The shift in terminology also typically signaled the need for increasing numbers of carefully worded objectives to specify the goals that had been indicated earlier by a smaller number of more loosely worded intentions. In this regard, the behavioral objectives movement is said to have collapsed under its own weight. (pp. 117–118)

I am certain students feel this weight when being confronted by a long list of objectives that, while designed with good intentions, were, nevertheless, overwhelming instead of instructive.

To me, this approach, although well accepted in the nursing community, does not take into consideration the complexities of nursing practice and supports teaching in the fragmented, decontextualized manner that has plagued nursing education for decades and may obstruct the realization of transforming nursing education, the path that Benner and her colleagues (1984/2010) have outlined. Thus, I believe the time has come to rethink how we write objectives, and how we communicate desired outcomes to students.

RETHINKING OBJECTIVES TO TRANSFORM NURSING EDUCATION

What I propose is a change in definitions and the way we think about goals, objectives, and outcomes. To support the learning outcomes that will truly transform nursing education, the outcomes we share with students should be broadly written and encompass complex performance and abilities. Consequently, objectives should be written more broadly like a goal, but in the format suggested by Mager (1997), which includes a description of the performance, a broad condition, and a criterion when appropriate. Although speaking from the perspective of medicine, Harden's (2002) perspective is that objectives are really learning outcomes or goals that:

- Are user friendly and not too cumbersome and can be readily adopted by teachers and students
- Highlight the key broad learning outcomes
- Take account of the realities of medical practice where knowledge, skills, and attitudes are integrated to make up competences
- Engage the individual teacher and student and give them some measure of ownership of the process (pp. 154–155)

Identifying Learning Outcomes

To begin the process of writing objectives, I recommend thinking in terms of the broad *learning outcomes* that should be met by the end of the course. Start thinking about this by writing: *At the end of this course, I want students to . . .* and complete the sentence with a bulleted list. Write down what comes to mind without editorial comments by that regulatory inner voice. Refining can be done later. Keep in mind that from a constructivist perspective, the contents of this list may actually be broad enough to become objectives. All that is needed are measurable verbs.

Questions to consider as you think about desired learning outcomes are:

1. What content is unique to this course?
2. What knowledge, skills, and attitudes must students take away from this course because it is not included in any other?

Be sure to include in this initial list of outcomes any *programmatic* outcomes that must be achieved. Reflecting on a few additional questions can be helpful, such as:

- How and where does this course fit into the broader curriculum for the program?
- Are there terminal program outcomes that students must meet, the content for which comes from this course?
- Does this course provide foundational content for which some facts must be memorized and understanding achieved, or is this a course in which students apply previously learned knowledge?
- What is the requisite knowledge that must be revisited and built into contextualized learning?

BOX 4.6
SAMPLE LIST OF LEARNING OUTCOMES

At the end of the course, I want students to:

- Activate prior knowledge from the basic science courses, such as anatomy and physiology and pathophysiology, and associate them with physical assessment
- Learn how to obtain a comprehensive and focused history by asking branching questions to pursue a line of inquiry
- Learn to extract the salient information on the history to guide what systems are assessed on the exam
- Learn *the moves*, such as where to place the stethoscope to hear S4 or right-middle-lobe lung sounds
- Learn when and why to use specific and specialized assessment techniques such as egophony, for example, when lung sounds seem diminished in a lung base
- Learn to distinguish normal from abnormal findings
- Learn to integrate multiple findings and associate them with a specific pathology to validate or refute information obtained on the history and arrive at a diagnosis or list of plausible diagnoses

For example, in a health (or physical) assessment course, learning is complex and proceeds down several pathways. Box 4.6 demonstrates a list of outcomes that could be written. These are broad outcomes written with verbs that are not measurable. They indicate learning that is not content-specific, which in a health assessment course means body system–specific. Measuring or assessing specific objectives written for each body system would be too time consuming, increase cognitive load for students, and is related to what I consider the old paradigm of objective writing.

Translating Broad Goals to Broad Objectives

Because the desired outcome from a constructivist perspective is integration of these skills, the objectives should reflect that. If specific, focused objectives are written for every body system to reflect the outcomes listed in Box 4.6, a large list will result. Consider an objective that reads: *At the end of the course, the student will be able to distinguish* (comprehension level, cognitive domain) *normal from pathologic heart sounds to arrive at a diagnosis.* The desired outcome of this objective can be incorporated into a more broadly written one that will assess other subordinate skills as well. An objective that states the desired global outcome might be: *At the end of the course, the student will be able to compile a list of plausible diagnoses based on elements of the history and normal and abnormal findings on physical examination.* The verb "compile" is from the cognitive domain, synthesis level—a high-level verb. Indicating that this is the desired level of learning is consistent with (a) an integrated constructivist approach, (b) the use of higher cognitive skills, (c) the ability to assess multiple systems under the guise of one objective, and (d) the choice of a wide range of assessment strategies.

Perhaps, the question in your mind now is how will students understand exactly what they need to learn to meet the objective? To answer that, an understanding of the affordances of the online environment is needed. Although this topic will be discussed in greater detail in subsequent chapters, online multiple-choice quizzes can point out important knowledge and understandings from the assigned readings with questions building to application, analysis, synthesis, and evaluation. Questions based on a case will help students anchor what they are learning in an appropriate context. Quizzes of this nature accompany each content area (weekly or biweekly), are formative in nature, can be taken multiple times to achieve mastery, and are worth only a few points so students take the learning content seriously. In addition, a podcast to introduce each content area explaining to students why the information is important to their future role, the rationale for the quizzes, and an explanation for other assignments or assessments will help students focus their study time.

The outcomes for student learning at the RN to bachelor of science in nursing (BSN) or graduate level should focus on higher cognitive functions. The desired learning in each course should begin with students activating prior knowledge (what they know and understand) and associated relevant experiences. What they already know and understand is then reviewed in light of the new role-specific content they are learning and their understanding is then validated, updated, or completely revised, resulting in a higher level of performance. Because the goal is an integration of many components of performance, global objectives should be written to align students' expectations for learning with faculty's expectations of performance. An example will be forthcoming, but first, additional background information must be discussed.

Process of Writing Broad Objectives—A Task Analysis

Once this list of learning outcomes or goals has been completed, an example of which is in Box 4.6, these statements can be converted to objectives. Keep in mind that while cognitive activity lives in the background of most affective and psychomotor performance, it is important to be clear about the *type of performance to be assessed* and to write an objective to communicate that. Thus, the first step is to determine the domain: cognitive, psychomotor, or affective. Once the domain has been chosen for an objective, the next step is to choose a level within that domain. From a constructivist perspective, the rule of thumb should be to aim for the highest level that is associated with the desired real-life performance. Questions to ask yourself that follow a logical sequence to help you build the objective are presented in Exhibit 4.5. Once you have written the objective, reread it to be certain that the sentence is in good form grammatically. As you can see after reviewing the questions, using the Backward Design method

EXHIBIT 4.5
Questions to Ask Yourself as You Build the Objective

To Determine	Questions to Ask
The domain	1. What is the desired type of learning involved—thinking (cognitive); muscle movement (psychomotor); or feelings attitudes, or values (affective)? *Keep in mind that cognitive processes lurk in the background of psychomotor and affective learning.* 2. How will the learning from this domain be assessed? 3. How will the content be taught?
Once a decision has been made as to the appropriate domain, the next step is to determine the desired level of learning within that domain.	
Level of learning (within the domain)	1. What level of learning or performance is required in order for the students to function in their future role? 2. How can this level of learning be *authentically* assessed? 3. Will that type of assessment indicate mastery as expected by the role? 4. How will this content be taught? *Jumping ahead in the Backward Design process to consider assessment strategies and teaching methods may help you determine the level of performance required.*
Verb	Which verb from the list associated with the domain and level chosen: 1. Best informs me of the desired performance, assessment, and teaching methods? 2. Expresses to students what is ultimately expected of them? 3. Makes the most sense from a grammatical and syntax perspective?
The outcome or goal, assessment, and teaching methods should be aligned with the domain, level, and verb chosen for the objective. If they are not aligned, repeat these steps.	

(Wiggins & McTighe, 2005) in every step of writing objectives will ensure that you have considered assessment and teaching methods when making decisions about the domain, level, and verb. Keep in mind as you are asking yourself these questions that you should not get hung up on assessments and teaching methods. Jot down ideas, but maintain focus on writing the objectives at the appropriate domain and appropriate level within that domain. Let us go through the steps of this process with an example.

To illustrate this process, it may be useful to complete a task analysis (Mager, 1997), a means to determine the components of learning required to meet the desired outcome. Returning to the advanced health assessment course, perhaps an identified outcome would be for students to be able to combine findings on the history and exam to arrive at a diagnosis. Successfully meeting this objective requires that students activate prior knowledge from their pathophysiology course and correlate it with findings on the history and exam. Although the learning required could be considered both cognitive and psychomotor, we will first focus on writing a cognitive objective. As the verb "correlate" comes to mind when thinking about what we want students to do, synthesis is involved, which means putting pieces of data together to create a unified and unique whole. A verb from the cognitive domain, synthesis level would be appropriate to describe the learning required. The objective arising from that desired outcome or goal might be: *At the end of the course, the student will be able to correlate salient information from the history with abnormal findings on a focused physical examination to arrive at a plausible diagnosis.* The verb correlate is from the synthesis level of Bloom's cognitive domain. Completing a task analysis on the objective will help you fully understand the component skills that must be mastered to meet this objective. The results of this process are shown in Box 4.7. Although the outcome of the task analysis looks very similar to the initial list of outcomes, the task analysis is more specific to the objective. For example, the objective is cognitive, so the ability to perform examination techniques is not relevant.

Getting ahead of things a bit, one can readily see how taking the time to complete a task analysis sets the stage for the development of a rubric that can be used to grade the performance. This topic is discussed in detail in Chapter 9, but suffice to say that a task analysis is a worthwhile activity, done early on to fully understand the components that go into the performance to validate that you will be assessing what you wanted to assess.

The take-away point here is to aim as high as possible when choosing a verb for an objective. Consider at the least the application-level verbs and *above* in the cognitive domain; the "receiving" through "organization" levels in the affective domain; and the "guided response" level and *below* in the psychomotor domain. Remember to start the list of objectives with

---

BOX 4.7
SAMPLE TASK ANALYSIS OF AN OBJECTIVE

- Ask appropriate questions on the history
- Extract the salient data from the information obtained in the history
- Based on the salient data, determine what systems should be assessed on exam
- Know which basic and specialized examination techniques are indicated
- Know what the normal findings are for the examination techniques used
- Recognize an abnormal finding and what it indicates
- Understand how the findings on exam validate or refute what was found on the history
- Combine the data to arrive at a plausible diagnosis

---

the condition: *At the end of the course the student will be able to (or can)* and a criterion if appropriate. Another rule of thumb is to keep the number of objectives to fewer than 10; including six is really more practical. The reasoning behind this recommendation is that (a) too many objectives can increase cognitive load and be overwhelming for students; (b) may indicate to faculty that either too much course content is planned for the course, or that faculty have not written broad objectives that truly assess authentic performance.

COMMON MISTAKES MADE WHEN WRITING OBJECTIVES

Writing objectives is not an easy task. Seasoned faculty often struggle with the process, mainly because they do not often write objectives. Most likely, their job is to interpret objectives provided by the curriculum committee in order to determine appropriate assessment methods and teaching strategies, topics discussed later in this chapter.

Common mistakes made when writing objectives are shown in Box 4.8.

Too Specific, Too Many, Too Narrow

The mistake of writing specific objectives in a step-wise fashion probably originated with Mager's (1997) early behaviorist-driven ideas of writing objectives in a step-wise fashion that reflected the order in which content

---

BOX 4.8
COMMON MISTAKES MADE WHEN WRITING OBJECTIVES

- Are too specific and written in a step-wise fashion
- Are not broadly written to reflect the complexity of performance necessary for the role
- Are focused on process and not outcomes; on teaching and not learning
- Include two verbs in one objective (two outcomes)
- Include verbs not appropriate for the domain that faculty plan to assess
- Include words and phrasing that are difficult to understand

---

was taught. This is problematic on two fronts. First, objectives should state desired learning outcomes and be written from the student's perspective (Bloom, 1956; Gronlund, 1995; Mager, 1997). Recall that the recommended condition is: *At the end of the course, the **student** will be able to . . .*, which indicates that what follows will be a broad statement of performance that combines multiple sublayers of learning acquired throughout the course. Second, all objectives must be assessed. Writing multiple specific objectives takes the focus away from the desired integration of concepts and requires instead assessing the individual elements of content taught.

Process Instead of Outcome

Writing objectives that describe a process instead of an outcome is easy to do. For example, the verb "discuss" is often included in lists of verbs for the comprehension level of the cognitive domain. As discussion boards are often used in online courses, this verb seems appropriate. However, it describes the *process* in which knowledge construction occurs, not the outcome. If students discuss a topic, but they are off base on many aspects of the content, do they meet the objective? The best way to avoid writing process-oriented objectives is to be clear on the learning outcomes before starting to write your objectives.

Two Verbs

By far, the most common mistake encountered is including two measurable verbs in one objective. This indicates a poor understanding of a taxonomy. Remember that a taxonomy in educational terms is a hierarchy of learning that proceeds from simple to complex and concrete to the abstract in the cognitive domain (Bloom, 1956), integration in the affective domain (Krathwohl et al., 1964), and increasing fluidity and automaticity of movement in the psychomotor domain (Simpson, 1966). For example, consider the objective: *At the end of the course, the student will be able to use appropriate physical examination techniques and discriminate normal from abnormal findings on a focused physical examination to arrive at a diagnosis.* Two measurable cognitive domain verbs are included: "use" is from the application level and "discriminate" is from the analysis level (Gronlund, 1995). When the necessary cognitive skills are considered for this performance, it seems obvious that one must recall (knowledge level) appropriate examination techniques, understand (comprehension) what they indicate, be able to use (application level) these techniques correctly in a given situation in order to elicit findings and discriminate (analysis level) normal from abnormal. From the hierarchy of learning represented in the taxonomy, one cannot discriminate findings unless one has the necessary requisite skills. The lower cognitive activity is subsumed in the higher. So, the application-level verb "use" is unnecessary, as this skill was learned in order to perform at a higher level. The assessment chosen must assess the student's ability to discriminate, which by default also assesses the lower cognitive levels.

Using two verbs in one objective is problematic from another perspective. If a student meets the performance requirements indicated by one verb and not the other, did the student meet the objective? This argues against using verbs from two different levels of the same or different domains in one objective. Consider this objective: *At the end of the course, the student will be able to explain why assessing specific systems was indicated by the history and perform an appropriate, history-guided focused physical examination.* Here, a verb, "explain" (cognitive domain, comprehension level), and a second verb, "perform" (psychomotor domain, complex overt response level), are used in the same objective. If students cannot explain why they chose to examine a specific system, yet flawlessly perform the focused exam, did they meet the objective? So the question to ask is, could students have completed an *appropriate* exam without understanding why they were doing so?

Verbs in Multiple Domains

Many lists of measurable verbs are available on the Internet and in nursing texts. In some of these lists, the same verb appears in more than one domain, requiring that when writing objectives you first become clear on the type of performance required (the domain). Let us look at this objective as an example: *At the end of the course, the student will be able to discriminate normal from abnormal findings on a focused physical examination.* The verb "discriminate" can be found in two domains in some lists of verbs for objectives

(Bastable & Alt, 2014): in the analysis level of the cognitive domain and the guided response mechanism and complex overt response levels of the psychomotor domain. Let us assume that you plan to assess this objective by having the student complete a focused history and physical examination on a standardized patient and verbally present the case to you. Is this a cognitive or psychomotor performance that is being assessed? Although performance involves using the correct assessment techniques of inspection, auscultation, percussion, and/or palpation, which are cognitive and psychomotor skills, what the objective is really about is *discriminating normal from abnormal findings*, which is a cognitive activity. True, the techniques of performing a physical examination that students use during the exam with the standardized patient can be observed and faculty will make some decisions whether the techniques were performed correctly, but that is not what the objective is about. The objective will be assessed when the student presents the case. That is when you will be able to determine if the student identified and made a judgment based on abnormal findings.

Verb Does Not Match Desired Outcome

Another common mistake when writing objectives is using a verb from one domain to write an objective from another. Consider the following objective written to guide learning from a reflective journal: *At the end of the course, the student will be able to recall feelings and attitudes after completing a visit with a dying patient.* The verb "recall" is used in two domains: the cognitive domain at the knowledge level and the affective domain at the responding level (Bastable & Alt, 2014). Because feelings and attitudes are the focus of the affective domain, what will be assessed by this objective is the student's ability to later *recall* (knowledge level, cognitive domain) the feelings at the time of the encounter, which is a *cognitive* activity. If the objective were: *At the end of the course the student will be able to express* (organization level of the affective domain) *understanding and empathy of the dying patient through body language, reassuring words, or silence,* assessing performance in the affective domain could be done by observing the student interacting with a dying patient.

Gibberish

In an effort to sound scholarly, some faculty write objectives that are very difficult to understand because of the words chosen, the convoluted sentence structure, or incomprehensible terms, something that Mager (1997) refers to as "gibberish" (p. 142). Mager cites this example: "Embark on a lifelong search for truth, with the willingness and ability to pose questions, examine experience, and construct explanations and meanings" (p. 143). Not only is the verb "embark" not measurable, but from a student's perspective it would also be difficult to understand what performance is required to successfully meet the objective. This pitfall can be avoided by keeping in mind that the purpose of objectives is to communicate the desired performance to students so they can adequately prepare for the assessment. Keeping language simple and using an economy of words will ensure that all stakeholders understand the objectives.

TRANSLATING PROVIDED OBJECTIVES

Often in academia, course objectives are written by the curriculum committee and cannot be changed by faculty who will be teaching the course. Although this seems to somewhat restrict academic freedom, the curriculum committee has the broad programmatic overview required to assign learning outcomes to courses throughout the program, thereby avoiding unnecessary repetition of content and ensuring that content required to function in the particular nursing role and by accrediting bodies is included. The job for faculty becomes devising assessments and teaching strategies to ensure that students actually learn what they are expected to learn to meet the objectives. A useful step in coming to terms with provided objectives is to complete a task analysis of the objective as was discussed in an earlier section, Process of Writing Broad Objectives—A Task Analysis.

COURSE-ALIGNMENT TEMPLATES

Although the focus of this chapter has been on writing goals and objectives, I have mentioned how this activity must be aligned with assessment strategies and teaching methods. To help you keep the entire process in mind, I developed two course-alignment templates that follow the Backward Design process of Wiggins and McTighe (2005). Exhibit 4.6 can be used when

EXHIBIT 4.6
Course-Alignment Template for Use When Writing Objectives

Outcomes	Objectives—*At the End of This Course, the Students Will Be Able to:*	Assessments	Teaching Strategies

EXHIBIT 4.7
Course-Alignment Template for Use When Interpreting Objectives

Course description:
Objectives:

Objective Number	Assessments	Teaching Strategies

Note: See the Appendix for a template that can be downloaded for interactive use.

you are tasked with writing the objectives for a course. In this exhibit, the outcomes or goals appear in the far-left column, followed by columns for the objectives, assessments, and teaching strategies. Exhibit 4.7 can be used when the objectives have been written for you and your job is to identify the appropriate assessments and teaching strategies that align. These numbered objectives, and perhaps the course description as well, should be copied and pasted at the top of this exhibit to keep you focused. The columns in this exhibit are listed in the following order: objective number, assessments, and teaching strategies.

Most likely you will assess each objective in multiple ways. For example, you may plan a quiz with each module to take advantage of the testing effect discussed in Chapter 1. In the course-alignment template, you can list the quizzes by number and the actual discussion questions as well. Keep in mind that in online teaching, formative and summative assessments as well as some of the teaching methods may be the same activity. This is also discussed in detail in Chapter 1.

THE TAKE-AWAY

Course objectives remain useful for faculty when designing an online course and for students as a road map toward learning. However, if we are to transform nursing education that integrates didactic and clinical practice, *knowing that* with *knowing how* within an authentic context, and ways of thinking that go beyond critical thinking, our objectives must be globally written, perhaps a new paradigm in writing course objectives. To help with the process, a task analysis of the performance as well as consideration of potential assessments and teaching methods are helpful. A task analysis of the objective, once written, is a way of validating that the performance is accurately specified within the objective.

REFERENCES

Anderson, L. W. (2003). Benjamin S. Bloom: His life, his works, and his legacy. In B. J. Zimmerman & Dale H. Schunk (Eds.), *Educational psychology: A century of contributions* (pp. 367–389). Mahwah, NJ: Lawrence Erlbaum.

Anderson, L. W., & Sosniak, L. A. (Eds.). (1994). *Bloom's taxonomy: A forty-year retrospective.* Ninety-third yearbook of the National Society for the Study of Education, Part 2. Chicago, IL: University of Chicago Press.

Bastable, S. B., & Alt, M. F. (2014). Behavioral objectives. In S. B. Bastable (Ed.), *Nurse as educator: Principles of teaching and learning for nursing practice* (4th ed., pp. 423–468). Burlington, MA: Jones & Bartlett.

Benner, P. (1984/2001). *From novice to expert: Excellence and power in clinical nursing practice.* Upper Saddle River, NJ: Prentice Hall Health. (Commemorative edition. Original work published 1984)

Benner, P., Sutphen, M., Leonard, V., & Day, L. (1984/2010). *Educating nurses: A call for radical transformation.* San Francisco, CA: Jossey-Bass.

Bloom, B. S. (1956). *The taxonomy of educational objectives, the classification of educational goals: Handbook I.* New York, NY: David McKay.

Dave, R. (1970). *Psychomotor levels in developing and writing objectives.* Tucson, AZ: Educational Innovators Press.

Felder, R. M., & Brent, R. (1997). Objectively speaking. *Chemical Engineering Education, 31*(3), 178–179.

Forrest, S. P., III, & Peterson, R. O. (2006). It's called andragogy. *Academy of Management Learning & Education, 5*(1), 113–122.

Greeno, J. G. (1976). Cognitive objectives of instruction: Theory of knowledge for solving problems and answering questions. In D. Klahr (Ed.), *Cognition and instruction* (pp. 123–159). Hillsdale, NJ: Lawrence Erlbaum.

Gronlund, N. E. (1995). *How to write and use instructional objectives* (5th ed.). Englewood Cliffs, NJ: Merrill.

Harden, R. M. (2002). Learning outcomes and instructional objectives: Is there a difference? *Medical Teacher, 24*(2), 151–155.

Harrow, A. J. (1972). *A taxonomy of the psychomotor domain: A guide for developing behavioral objectives.* New York, NY: David McKay.

Krathwohl, D. R. (2002). A revision of Bloom's taxonomy: An overview. *Theory Into Practice, 41*(4), 212–218.

Krathwohl, D. R., Bloom, B. S., & Masia, B. B. (1964). *The taxonomy of educational objectives, the classification of educational goals: Handbook II.* New York, NY: David McKay.

Lalley, J. P., & Gentile, J. R. (2009). Adapting instruction to individuals: Based on the evidence, what should it mean? *International Journal of Teaching and Learning in Higher Education, 20*(3), 462–475.

Mager, R. F. (1997). *Preparing instructional objectives: A critical tool in the development of effective instruction* (3rd ed.). Atlanta, GA: Center for Effective Performance Press.

Marken, J., & Morrison, G. (2013). Objectives over time: A look at four decades of objectives in the educational research literature. *Contemporary Educational Technology, 4*(1), 1–14.

Martin, B. L., & Reigeluth, C. M. (1999). Affective education and the affective domain: Implications for instructional-design theories and models. In C. M. Reigeluth (Ed.), *Instructional-design theories and models, volume II: A new paradigm of instructional theory* (pp. 485–509). Mahwah, NJ: Lawrence Erlbaum.

Mayer, R. E. (1998). Cognitive, metacognitive, and motivational aspects of problem-solving. *Instructional Science, 26*, 49–63.

Merriam, S. B., & Leahy, B. (2005). Learning transfer: A review of the research in adult education and training. *PAACE Journal of Lifelong Learning, 14*, 1–24.

Oermann, M. H. (1990). Psychomotor skill development. *Journal of Continuing Education in Nursing, 21*(5), 202–204.

Oermann, M. H., & Gaberson, K. B. (2014). *Evaluation and testing in nursing education* (4th ed.). New York, NY: Springer Publishing.

Reilly, D. E., & Oermann, M. H. (1985). *The clinical field: Its use in nursing education.* Norwalk, CT: Appleton-Century-Crofts.

Reynolds, R. E., Sinatra, G. M., & Jetton, T. L. (1996). Views of knowledge acquisition and representation: A continuum from experience centered to mind centered. *Educational Psychologist, 31*(2), 93–104.

Simpson, E. J. (1966). *The classification of educational objectives, psychomotor domain* [VTE OE 5-85-104]. Washington, D C: U.S. Department of Health, Education, and Welfare, Education Office.

Sosniak, L. A. (1994). The taxonomy, curriculum and their relations. In L. W. Anderson & L. A. Sosniak (Eds.), *Bloom's taxonomy: A forty-year retrospective.* Ninety-third yearbook of the National Society for the Study of Education, *Part 2*. Chicago, IL: University of Chicago Press.

Sylvester, R. (1995). *A celebration of neurons: An educator's guide to the human brain.* Alexandria, VA: Association for Supervision and Curriculum Development.

Tanner, C. A. (2006). Thinking like a nurse: A research-based model of clinical judgment in nursing. *Journal of Nursing Education, 45*(6), 204–211.

Wiggins, G., & McTighe, J. (2005). *Understanding by design* (2nd ed.). Alexandria, VA: Association for Supervision and Curriculum Development.

Wilson, B. G., & Myers, K. M. (2000). Situated cognition in theoretical and practical context. In D. H. Johassen & S. M. Land (Eds.), *Theoretical foundations of learning environments* (pp. 57–88). Mahwah, NJ: Lawrence Erlbaum.

Zul, J. E. (2002). *The art of changing the brain: Enriching the practice of teaching by exploring the biology of the brain.* Sterling, VA: Stylus.

5

Rethinking Teaching and Assessments

TRANSFORMING NURSING EDUCATION

In their call for radical transformation in nursing education, a must read for all nurse educators, Benner, Sutphen, Leonard, and Day (1984/2010) made four recommendations to accomplish the "integration of knowledge, skilled know-how, and ethical comportment" (p. 82) when educating nurses. These recommendations call for nurse educators to:

- "Teach for a sense of salience, situated cognition, and action in particular situations" (p. 82)
- Integrate classroom and clinical teaching
- Emphasize clinical reasoning and multiple ways of thinking that include critical thinking
- Emphasize formation instead of socialization to the role

Although the site visits that provided the information for their book were done in undergraduate programs of nursing exclusively, eight generic and one RN to bachelor of science in nursing (BSN) program, their findings apply to graduate nursing education as well. Discussing these recommendations in more detail, you will understand how they are grounded in sound educational theory and provide a framework to improve our teaching.

The first recommendation is in reaction to teaching decontextualized content organized in textbook fashion such that students' only choice was to memorize. Content is presented in such courses as lists of isolated facts and categorized information with little indication of how to use this information. Without applying it to a specific patient's situation, students cannot extract the important or salient information, understand why it is so, and use it to guide practice. As Brown, Collins, and Duguid (1989) note:

> in order to learn these subjects (and not just to learn about them) students need much more than abstract concepts and self-contained examples.

> They need to be exposed to the use of a domain's conceptual tools in authentic activity—to teachers acting as practitioners and using these tools in wrestling with problems of the world. (p. 34)

This authentic context provides a backdrop for the theory of situated cognition (Lave & Wenger, 1991) in which learning is enhanced when cognitive activities are embedded in a real-life context of co-participation. Foundational to situated cognition is that *knowing* cannot be separated from *doing*, and by giving students opportunities to wrestle with problems common to the role that are complex and unstable, students learn to recognize what is important and what is not when assessing a situation and problem solving. This is what Benner et al. (1984/2010) referred to when they encouraged nurse educators to teach for a *sense of salience*, or "linking perception and discernment with the ability to use knowledge from a rich knowledge base" (p. 83).

The second recommendation focuses on the separation of classroom and clinical teaching, which applies to online teaching as well. During the site visits that were the basis for their conclusions, Benner et al. (1984/2010) noticed that although students had adequate time to practice skills in a skills lab, for example, doing so was not embedded in a case scenario representing a real-life situation, again referring to the separation of knowing and doing from a relevant context. From an online teaching perspective, lectures are not the main teaching method as they often are in the classroom. Instead, small group discussions become the learning space. Creating engaging discussion questions (DQs), the topic of Chapter 7, allows for the combination of theory and application, content and context.

In the third recommendation, Benner et al. (1984/2010) referred to the term *critical thinking*, which they feel has become a "catch all phrase" (p. 84) when referring to the various cognitive processes that nurses use to problem solve. They point to the broader need for nursing students to develop skillful critical reflection, clinical and diagnostic reasoning, and "creative, scientific, and formal criterial reasoning" (p. 85) processes. However, what can be taught directly is the theory of these cognitive processes only, which results in knowing. Students then need the opportunity to develop these cognitive skills through practice using these skills (doing) when problem solving in real-life situations without the chance of hurting anyone.

To the online nursing educator, *doing* refers to using cognitive skills and is best promoted by teaching content within context, either engaging DQs or authentic cases. Although students may know the definition of diagnostic reasoning and the steps of the process, unless they apply that knowledge to a case situation, they are really not doing diagnostic reasoning.

Online discussions provide such opportunities, if the questions asked require higher cognitive functioning. Fact-based questions, the answers to which can easily be found in a textbook, will not suffice, yet this is what frequently occurs in online discussions. This not only results in little mean-ingful discussion, but also in repetitive answers as students struggle to post something that has not already been said. Fact-based questions can increase cognitive load (Chapter 1) when only one correct answer exists. *Ill-structured* and *messy* cases that mimic the complex nature of actual nursing practice are necessary to combine theory and practice and allow students to test the waters of the role or do the type of thinking required by the role. How to create ill-structured cases is the topic of Chapter 6.

In addition to and in order for students to use these cognitive skills effectively, developing metacognitive skills is necessary. Recall that meta-cognition is the executive control and regulation one has over cognition, or thinking. Although the term *metacognition* is often used interchangeably with *reflection,* reflection activities are often *assigned* in nursing as a means to encourage students to review something that occurred in the past. This is different from metacognition, in my view. Although both processes require *thinking,* the type of reflection often required of students is reflection-*on*-action, which occurs long after the fact. Metacognition, on the other hand, exerts control over problem solving during the problem-solving activity itself, guiding thinking to consider multiple perspectives and to question understanding (Pintrich, 2002). It is more consistent with Schön's (1983) view of reflection-*in*-action, yet this term is seldom heard. Metacognition is the vehicle that sets critical thinking or habits of thought in motion and is a skill that can be learned.

The final recommendation is for nurse educators to expand their focus on socialization to nursing practice and the nursing role to that of forma-tion. The term *formation* means the process of being formed or "to being constituted by the meanings, content, intents, and practice of nursing rather than merely learning or being socialized into a nursing role in an external way" (Benner et al., 1984/2010, pp. 86–87). Again the authors reiterate the need for this formation to occur in an authentic context. By placing the stu-dents in the role they aspire to through messy online case discussions, they begin to think like a professional nurse, for the RN–BSN student, and like a nurse practitioner, educator, administrator, or researcher, for the gradu-ate nurse. Here, modeling and coaching of the role by faculty during these discussions is of utmost importance.

IMPLEMENTING THE RECOMMENDATIONS

Teaching Content Within Context

What these four recommendations have in common is *teaching in con-text,* or situated in real-life scenarios, similar to clinical experiences. This concept was discussed in Chapter 2 in the Situated Cognition section, but is so central to creating engaging online teaching and assessment methods that it is reviewed here. Thus, when creating authentic contexts, we want the scenarios to be true to the specific experiences students will encounter in the role they aspire to. Also important to consider, as we plan for changing the way we teach, is that assessment drives learning (Beattie, Collins, & McInnes, 1997), so the assessments we choose must be congruent with how we teach. Consequently, meeting the call to radical transformation in our teaching will require authentic assessments and authentic teaching methods.

Although the call to transform nursing education and the changes necessary to accomplish this are clearly outlined in these recommendations, operationalizing them has been a challenge for multiple reasons, one of which, I believe, is faculty lacking the know-how. The goal of this chapter is to introduce the notion that teaching methods and assessments are one and the same in online education if (a) the context for learning is *authentic*, a term that is reviewed in the next section, Authentic Defined, and (b) the questions asked require higher cognitive functioning to answer.

Authentic Defined

One definition of *authentic* can be something that is real or genuine, not copied or false; that is, true and accurate. Recall from Chapter 2 that situated cognition, a sociocultural learning theory, first introduced the importance of teaching content in context, and it is what Benner et al. (1984/2010) are referring to in their first recommendation, listed at the beginning of this chapter. In education, an authentic context is defined by its characteristics, which are listed in Box 5.1.

The most common teaching methods that meet the criterion of authentic include open-ended, ill-structured DQs, case-based DQs, case studies, unfolding cases, and problem-based learning (PBL). Creating authentic DQs is discussed in Chapter 7 and writing cases is discussed in Chapter 6. Any type of scenario or story that presents a realistic, complex problem or dilemma to be solved or a goal to be achieved that sets the stage for student collaboration in small groups will meet the criteria for authenticity. These types of teaching strategies create context if essential elements are present.

Ill Structured Defined

In addition to providing an authentic context, ill-structured or ill-defined or messy cases, as they are also referred to in the educational literature, are

---

BOX 5.1
AUTHENTIC DEFINED

In the educational context as defined by Herrington, Reeves, and Oliver (2010), authentic means to:

- Provide authentic contexts that reflect the way the knowledge will be used in real life
- Provide authentic tasks
- Provide access to expert performance and the modeling of processes
- Provide multiple roles and perspectives
- Support collaborative construction of knowledge
- Promote reflection to enable abstractions to be formed
- Promote articulation to enable tacit knowledge to be made explicit
- Provide coaching and scaffolding by the teacher at critical times
- Provide authentic assessment of learning within the tasks

Source: Herrington, Reeves, and Oliver (2010, p. 18). Used with permission from Dr. J. Herrington.

---

used to generate discussion and require the type of thinking that Benner et al. (1984/2010) describe as "multiple ways of thinking, such as clinical reasoning, and clinical imagination as well as critical, creative, scientific, and formal criterial reasoning" (p. 85). Problems in real life, especially in nursing practice, are inherently messy in that information that is relevant, irrelevant, and simply unnecessary is available simultaneously, and it is the nurse's job to extract the salient data, and use the higher cognitive functions of analysis, synthesis, and evaluation in order to formulate a plan and act.

Barrows and Kelson (1996, para. 25–47) list the essential elements of PBL problems that can be applied to any authentic teaching method (see Box 5.2). Cases or DQs with these characteristics evoke emotions that aid memory (Miller, 2014), are motivating for students, develop the thought processes important for the role, and promote transfer (Norman & Schmidt, 1992).

TEACHING AND ASSESSING AS ONE

Recall from Chapter 3 that the reconceptualized view of Wiggins and McTighe's (2005) Backward Design process for course development combined determining evidence that the outcomes had been met with choosing learning experiences and teaching methods into one step.

BOX 5.2
ESSENTIAL ELEMENTS OF PROBLEM-BASED LEARNING (PBL)

PBL cases:

- Are compelling, real-world situations
- Generate multiple viable hypotheses
- Stretch creative thinking
- Require knowledge
- Draw students toward curricular knowledge and skills
- Are designed to support inquiry
- Provide information only as requested
- Demand accountability
- Define the role for the student
- Incorporate a product or performance

However, can all assessments be used to teach? Although this idea will require a reconceptualization of assessment, I would answer "yes." The characteristics of assessments that double as methods of teaching include:

- Opportunities for formative feedback
- Multiple ways of thinking
- Timing in the course
- Relationship to desired learning outcomes

In addition, looking at the recommendations from Benner and colleagues (1984/2010), I would add that these methods are authentic and combine knowing that with knowing how and knowing when. So, basically what I am saying is that given the right framework, any assessment can be used to teach. However, in order to maintain the focus on assessing the desired course outcomes, first consider the best methods to assess the objectives and then consider how these methods can also be used to teach.

The process to determine the appropriate assessments and teaching methods begins with a review of the behavioral objectives for the course in order to ground future plans within the prescribed (from the curriculum committee) or faculty-determined learning outcomes. If the objectives have not been written, then doing so becomes the first step. Chapter 4 outlines the objective writing process. If the objectives have been provided, keep in mind that faculty cannot change them. Doing so requires approval from the curriculum committee, and oftentimes the entire faculty must vote on any changes.

Recall that the domain and level of verb used in the objective determines the level, but perhaps not the type of assessment. Verbs from the cognitive domain of Bloom's taxonomy—the application level and higher—are suitable for authentic DQs or case-based learning, either in small group discussions or as the basis for multiple-choice questions (MCQs) on a test. Those written at the lower cognitive levels, knowledge and comprehension, should be assessed with questions that require recall (fill in the blank) or recognition of the content (straightforward MCQs). Note that the knowledge and comprehension levels of Bloom's taxonomy are not consistent with combining knowing and doing as both levels are about knowing. Although skills assessment based on psychomotor or affective-domain verbs is typically done through simulation, role-playing, or demonstrations—an observation of students' performance by faculty—high-level DQs and case-based small group discussions that begin with a video clip of the patient or other stakeholder are particularly well suited to assessing objectives written in the affective domain.

Once the level of assessment required by the objectives is understood, the key question becomes: *How will meeting these outcomes play out in the students' future role?* This question will serve to maintain focus on the desired learning outcomes and specific understandings students must acquire as course planning continues. The ideal situation is for students to learn by wrestling with real-world problems that connect specific content in the course and prior knowledge to their future role. If they are given the opportunity to *think like a* _____ (fill in the blank with the student's desired role), what they are learning will be encoded in long-term memory as *cases* in a similar fashion to how it will be retrieved, thus making retrieval easier when the information is needed in practice. To accomplish this, authentic teaching methods situated in real-life contexts that combine knowing (content) and doing (skillful manipulation of that content and the habits of thought of the role) that promote collaborative constructivist learning can be used as the foundation for both teaching and learning. This can be accomplished with any content using cases or questions for discussion that mimic situations a student may encounter in the role.

The final aspect of assessment to consider is which assessments will be formative (assessment *for* learning) and which summative (assessment *of* learning). Again, most, if not all, types of assessment used in the online environment can be used for both. However, considering what is known from cognitive science research regarding the benefits of the testing effect and spaced study, the role of multiple-choice tests in learning and assessment has changed. Traditionally used as summative assessment in nursing education, their role as formative assessment and self-assessment is now well established.

Small group discussions have the potential for both formative and summative assessments if the DQ is ill structured, does not have one right answer, and requires students to employ multiple ways of thinking. To be used as formative assessment, faculty must be active in the discussion and provide feedback and guidance in order for students to meet the learning outcomes. Discussions of this type can subsequently be graded as summative assessment.

OPTIONS FOR ONLINE TEACHING AND ASSESSMENT

Given the research-based value of online group discussions, it is not surprising that they are included in the course design of most online nursing courses. A well-designed online course with authentic assessments and well-thought-out DQs is, by far, the best way to decrease faculty workload and make learning for students engaging and meaningful.

In a constructivist, learner-centered paradigm, learning should occur in a context that reflects how students will encounter the content, issues, or problems in their future roles. Ideally, this is done through group discourse in which knowledge is co-created with facilitation from faculty. The entire continuum from knowledge to evaluation in Bloom's cognitive domain, the affective domain, and the knowledge behind learning in the psychomotor domain can be learned within a context, such as that provided by a case study or well-written DQ. The discussions or assignments that fulfill these criteria are considered authentic.

Additional assignments appropriate for the online environment, such as quizzes or lessons to support if–then thinking, may be considered authentic, but this depends on how the questions are written. Quizzes can be used to support learning of knowledge and facts and, while useful to help scaffold learning, may not be considered authentic. These assignments can be used for either formative or summative assessment, or both. It depends on how they fit into your course design and the main purpose you have decided they will serve.

Small Group Discussions

Discussion boards are equivalent to classroom discussion, but hold additional benefits in that they allow time for reflection and composition of an evidence-based, well-thought-out response. They are also beneficial for shy or less verbal students, those who do not think fast on their feet, or who prefer not to speak up as they are afraid their responses will be incorrect. The benefit of online group discussions is that all students must participate and their responses can be objectively graded based on a rubric. Before deciding on the type of discussion to include in your course, it is important to consider the desired outcomes.

Pedagogical Benefits of Discussions

A misconception many faculty have, most likely held over from the days when lecture was used exclusively as the teaching method, is that students must be taught basic facts, concepts, and principles before they can apply them. Experience with PBL in the basic science courses during the initial 2 years of medical school has refined what is known about how and when students are capable of learning what. Medical students are a heterogeneous lot in that their educational preparation at the bachelor's level ranges from biology to business. Few are familiar with medical jargon, yet PBL is successful in engaging these students in the process of thinking like a physician and approaching problems with an inquisitive mind, taking responsibility for their learning. Although the *problem* presented may be a mystery to them initially, the *process* facilitated by an expert tutor encourages them to continually question what they really know and understand, identify what they need to learn to understand better and in greater depth, and the curiosity to find the answers. In other words, experience with case-based learning has brought to light that the lower levels of Bloom's taxonomy (knowledge, comprehension, and application) can be uncovered in the process of working through more complex cases requiring higher order thinking. Time need not be spent teaching facts, as students will inadvertently learn the basic information through independent study as they assimilate what they have read. The same is true for a non-case-based DQs. Perhaps Ross (1997) says it best when referring to problem-based curricula and how readings are not assigned; instead the task is for students to locate and evaluate what resources they need to work on the problem:

> This turns the normal approach to problem solving found in university and college programmes on its head. In the normal approach it is assumed that students have to have the knowledge required to approach a problem *before* they can start on the problem; here the knowledge arises *from work* on the problem. (p. 30)

Quizzes to Support Learning From Discussions

If faculty are concerned that students may not take the time to understand necessary facts, concepts, and principles, providing a multiple-choice quiz as formative assessment that focuses on the lower levels of Bloom's taxonomy is a better way to approach the acquisition of foundational knowledge. Students should be allowed to take these self-assessment quizzes worth minimal points multiple times in order to learn and understand basic information. This is also a means of preparing students for certification boards, which are typically MCQs. Also, if the questions are staged from knowledge through application where an incorrect answer becomes the upper border of their knowledge and ability, faculty can readily determine a specific point for remediation. In addition, quizzes of this type also point students to important content, which is helpful in situations in which readings include information beyond that which is essential for them to know and understand. Chapter 8 discusses writing quiz questions to achieve this.

Precursors to Successful Discussions

Grading Discussions

In order for discussions to be successful and to meet learning outcomes, a few preliminary decisions and actions by faculty are necessary. First, as discussions are where learning occurs, the learning spaces so to speak, value must be placed on them in terms of grades (Rovai, 2003).

How the discussions will be assessed and graded are decisions faculty must make early on before the course opens and the details are included in the syllabus. Sad to say, but discussions must be required and graded in order for students to contribute. In my experience, discussions that are optional will have minimal participation. The problem is that students do not have a sophisticated enough understanding of pedagogy to realize that knowledge is not only self-created, but co-created via discourse in a community set up for that purpose. Although grading and requirements for posting are really extrinsic motivators, they motivate students nevertheless.

Truthfully, I see grades as a hook to bring students into the discussions. If authentic questions or problems are posed, they will quickly find themselves engaged in the topic and process. And, if the relevance of the discussion topic is obvious to the student's future role, facilitating the discussion becomes much easier for faculty. Creating an engaging DQ is discussed in Chapter 7.

Expectations of Participation

Second, detailed expectations of students' participation and posting requirements must be clearly communicated, which should be included in the rubric to grade the discussions. My experience has found that adding this information to the syllabus is not enough. After the second week or so of classes, students seem to forget about the syllabus. Reminding them to look there creates another step students must complete to move on. While encouraging independence, that type of reminder often serves to frustrate students, as their interpretation is that you, as faculty, cannot take the time to answer their question. If this information is included in multiple places, such as in the discussion board link with the DQ and in the weekly announcement, and is consistently presented throughout the course, students will soon get into the rhythm of fulfilling posting requirements.

Logistics of Posting

Third, especially early on in the program, students may need specific directions of where and how to post. Although most likely your students are from the Net Generation (Gen-Xers or millennials), assuming they are tech savvy can cause unneeded frustration for both faculty and students. Posting directions as the course opens to avoid problems is imperative. This information should include:

- Where each discussion forum is located in the course
- What to click on within the discussion to create an initial post
- What to click on within the discussion to respond to a classmate's post
- How to change the subject line to reflect either the subject of the post or the student being replied to

Students are often embarrassed to ask questions about the logistics of posting as they think they should already know.

Discussion-Group Size

Group size for discussions of cases is a topic of debate. Baker (2011) indicated that groups of five to six students are sufficiently large for knowledge construction, but not so large that the number of posts becomes unwieldy. Palloff and Pratt (2003) advised that having fewer than five students in a group curbs interaction, and Rovai (2007) recommended that at least 10 students in each group were necessary to promote dialogue. In my experience, five is a good size—small enough for everyone to make a unique contribution without a great deal of overlap, without a large number of posts to read and digest.

Another less weighty decision regarding group formation is whether students will remain with the same group for each case or rotate in order to work with other students. Feedback I have received from students indicated that they preferred to stay in the same group in order to get to know a few students in the course well. I do feel this approach eliminates one variable or concern; that of becoming comfortable with a new group of students for each discussion, which may be especially difficult for shy, less assertive, or less confident students.

Logistical Decisions

Timing of Discussions

The first decision that needs to be made is the number of discussions you will have in the course. This is determined, to some degree, by the number of weeks in the course. However, the length of a discussion is important for learning. Weekly discussions do not allow enough time for students to learn in a deep, meaningful way. Online discussions should last 10 to 12 days, which is enough time for students to complete the necessary reading, synthesize what they have read, develop their initial post, and reply to classmates (Leppa, 2004). Starting the discussion on a Monday and ending it on a week from the following Friday (12 days later) will give students every other weekend without feeling they must monitor and participate in a discussion. Consider using these few days in between cases to have students reflect on what they have learned and the reasoning they have employed to reach conclusions, either as part of the discussion or in a personal journal. Some of the learning management systems (LMSs) include a journal feature that allows faculty to set up individual areas for students to reflect that can be seen only by the student and faculty.

Because each discussion will span almost 2 weeks, it is helpful to know the number of discussions the course can accommodate, considering holidays, required on-campus sessions, or midsemester breaks. If students are taking other courses concurrently, I recommend chatting with the other faculty to understand if any immersion sessions, residencies, or other on-campus meetings are required in their courses. Students will appreciate a lighter load the week they are on campus for anxiety-provoking assessments, face-to-face immersive learning experiences, or dissertation work with their committees. As the syllabus must be posted when the course opens, taking the time to consider the timing and number of discussions will ensure that an accurate syllabus is provided for students.

Expectations of Students in Discussions

When writing expectations of participation for students in discussions, be sure to include when the discussion will formally end in terms of grading and facilitation by faculty. In other words, if they decide to post on the weekend after the end date for the discussion, be sure it is understood whether those posts will be included as part of their grade and whether you will be active in the discussion during that time.

Programmatic Considerations

Additional considerations to assist you when actually writing the DQs are necessary such as understanding (a) where the course falls in the overall curriculum, that is, first semester, first year, and so on; (b) whether the courses in the program are sequenced such that all students follow the same path, that is, all students have taken the same courses; (c) whether students have already been exposed to this content before in their generic program or earlier in the program they are currently enrolled in; and (d) whether the course at hand is where they are to apply this previously encountered content, such as pathophysiology and pharmacology applied in a clinical course. Although it is understood that encountering the content does not mean it has been learned, it will give faculty a general idea of how complex the DQs can be.

Learning Management Set Up to Promote Learning

Another decision to make is whether students can view posts in other discussion groups or other students' posts within their group. Some LMSs, such as Moodle, can be set up so that each group cannot review another group's dialogue during the discussion, nor can a student see what his or her group mates have posted until posting for the first time. Because faculty want students to do their own work, blocking students from viewing the discussion until they post for the first time is ideal. Otherwise, students can develop a post based on what other students have said and not only avoid doing the necessary research, but also not engaging in critical, clinical, or diagnostic reasoning. Thus, the full value of discussions cannot be realized. Setting up an LMS to avoid issues with students not doing their own work can be a bit of a learning curve, but exploring this option is worthwhile.

VARIOUS TYPES OF DISCUSSIONS

Problem-Centered Discussions

Problem-centered discussions focus on a case, problem, issue, or dilemma that students will most likely encounter in their future roles. The goal of this type of discussion is to uncover (Wiggins & McTighe, 2005) prior knowledge as well as new understandings that are then applied to a specific real-life scenario. There is typically no one right answer to these cases, so students evaluate the evidence and arrive at a potential solution. This type of discussion promotes what Benner and colleagues (1984/2010) referred to as "multiple ways of thinking that includes critical thinking" (p. 84) as well as clinical and diagnostic reasoning, depending on the type of case. Problem-centered discussions are also an excellent means of promoting self-directed learning. When students encounter something they are unfamiliar with, they have the time to research it or ask questions. Case-based teaching and PBL are examples of problem-centered discussions. How to develop cases is the topic of Chapter 7. Developing engaging DQs around a commonly encountered problem, issue, or dilemma will also engage students and promote higher cognitive functioning. DQs that are authentic also promote coconstruction of knowledge, a valuable skill in nursing when dealing with today's complex health care environment. How to develop engaging discussions questions that are not case based is discussed in Chapter 6.

Project-Based Discussions

The term *project-based discussion* is not consistently defined in the literature. From my perspective, this type of discussion involves "asking learners to complete a project or work via collaborative discussion" (Wu, Hou, Hwang, & Liu, 2013, p. 63). Koh, Herring, and Hew (2010) and Wu et al. (2013) indicated that structured project-based discussions, those in which smaller assignments build to a final deliverable, seem to result in advanced levels of knowledge construction, perhaps due to formative feedback they receive on each stage of the project. This approach not only assures students that they are on the right track, but also allows time to make needed improvements prior to the final submission for a grade. The value for faculty is in staged grading, such as not having to grade large projects at the end of the semester only to find that students misinterpreted the assignment, were off track, or simply did not follow the guidelines.

The resulting deliverable of the project should be an authentic artifact—something useful to the student's future role. This might entail a plan to promote legislation, an evidence-based improvement project, a research proposal, or plan of care for a complex patient. Instead of writing a paper on the topic, students can present their product creatively via a YouTube video or PowerPoint presentation with speaker's notes, a Prezi, or Facebook page that not only lend themselves well to the virtual environment, but also teach valuable presentation skills that will serve them well in their future roles.

I would avoid asking students to write a group paper as the deliverable from a discussion. Unless the paper has been uploaded and edited in a wiki or GoogleDrive, faculty will not know what each team member's contribution was and if each student met the learning outcomes. Invariably, with a written product, one student is tasked with compiling everyone's contribution, which often entails rewriting the entire paper. I would also question the authenticity of this type of product. Although professional writing skills are important, demonstrating that is more in tune with an individual assignment.

Wu and colleagues (2013) included the term *collaborative* in their definition of project-based discussions. At this juncture, it is important to make a distinction between outcomes of a discussion that require *cooperation* as compared to *collaboration*. Although these terms are often considered synonymous, when applied to online discussions I see a difference. Misanchuk and Anderson (2001) considered cooperation akin to how a machine operates in that "different parts of the machine perform different functions and goals, but work together towards a similar end" (p. 7). Relating this to project-based or problem-centered online discussions, cooperative behavior occurs when students divide up the various aspects of a group project, work on them independently, and combine them in an assignment that is turned in as a deliverable. I have named this the *divide-and-conquer* approach, which seems to run contrary to constructivism and begs the question, how can students construct knowledge and form meaningful mental models if they learn only part of the whole? Students often take this approach in project-based discussions.

Misanchuk and Anderson described collaboration, on the other hand, as the group working together to achieve a goal, with students working on all aspects together. This type of approach will, most likely, result in the development of more complete mental models. This is the approach students typically take during a problem- or case-based discussion, even with a deliverable required at the end.

Morgan, Williams, Cameron, and Wade (2014) offered some very practical suggestions for implementing a project-based discussion. They are listed in Box 5.3 and include a few of my comments. If these suggestions are followed, participation is more likely to be equal and issues, few. Monitoring the discussion, intervening when necessary, and providing formative feedback on the assignments that build to the final project will help keep students on track.

Group Projects

Group projects differ from project-based discussions in that students typically start with an assigned topic or choose one from a list provided by faculty. The group then meets to create the group contract, assign roles, set a timeline, and determine how the project will be completed. This type of group work, common in face-to-face courses, has typically been done outside of the course with little faculty involvement, unless problems or questions arise within the group. The deliverable for group projects often is completed via the divide-and-conquer approach.

BOX 5.3
SUGGESTIONS FOR IMPLEMENTING A
PROJECT-BASED DISCUSSION

- Structure the task and provide guidelines and a timeline. I would add that having students turn in the project in stages for formative feedback is the best approach.
- Explain group roles. I would add here that an explanation of what collaboration means would be useful. This will avoid having students take the divide-and-conquer approach.
- Make group participation visible to faculty. I would add that having students conduct planning sessions in a discussion board or wiki is the best approach, although the unique benefit of a wiki is that students can edit the same document online. If students use different-colored fonts, you can easily see each student's contribution. Discourage face-to-face meetings even if that is geographically possible. Written summaries of these meetings add another layer of work for students and often do not reflect the participation from each member of the group.
- I recommend using GoogleDrive or Dropbox as a document repository for students to share reference materials. All members of the team can edit documents on GoogleDrive, so if a wiki is not available, this is a reasonable alternative. Both Dropbox and GoogleDrive are free and access can be restricted.

A separate grade should be awarded for participation leading to development of the deliverable from that of the deliverable itself. Students will appreciate the separation of process from product when it comes to being graded. This approach to grading will discourage the "free rider phenomenon of non-participating team members" (Wilson & Gerber, 2008, p. 34).

Group projects require that the group be autonomous and well functioning. Working within a group to achieve a goal teaches valuable non-content-related skills such as planning, sticking to a timeline, meeting deadlines, assuming various roles within the group, and resolving conflict. These skills are also valuable in the workplace. However, for nontraditional students, online group projects can be problematic depending upon work schedules, academic load, and time zones.

Recent research on how the millennials feel about group work is relevant here, even though it may be perpetuating stereotypes and implying they are a homogeneous bunch. The popular literature on the millennials seemed to indicate that they seek out groups in all facets of their lives (Howe & Strauss, 2000), including dating, working, and studying (Gurrie, 2015).

However, Gurrie's study involving 60 millennial students revealed that 82.8% preferred *not* to work in groups and 96.6% found themselves doing more than their share when they were involved in group work.

An interesting finding in the study by Walker et al. (2006) involving 134 millennial undergraduate nursing students revealed that their preferred method of learning was the lecture over group work, which may be due to recent exposure with the lecture method in secondary schools. Thus, when deciding whether to use a group project or engage students in a project-based discussion, I recommend carefully identifying the learning outcomes and weighing the pros and cons of this format.

If group work will help meet the learning outcomes, Wilson and Gerber (2008) stressed that millennials like structure and stability in course work. For that reason, I would recommend implementing the guidelines from Koh and colleagues (2010) listed in Box 5.4 when planning online group work that results in a product. To this I would add the recommendation of Morgan et al. (2014) to make student's individual contribution to group work visible by having students do the necessary planning in a discussion board, wiki, or GoogleDrive. This will allow you to grade each student's individual contribution separately from the product of the group's work, appealing to the millennials' need for recognition (Wilson & Gerber, 2008). The same types of deliverables as mentioned in the Project-Based Discussions section are appropriate for group projects.

Group work that results in a product can be beneficial and problematic when done online. Nontraditional students have constraints placed on their study time by work and family responsibilities. Because most of our students

---

BOX 5.4
GUIDELINES WHEN PLANNING GROUP WORK

- Assign a problem. The problem should be relevant to the members' future role and require discourse to discuss alternatives, resources, and potential solutions.
- Provide structure by breaking the final product into smaller stages that students turn in at regular intervals for feedback. This will support learning.
- Require a final, polished product in whatever medium students choose to help them create a complete mental model of what they have learned.
- Facilitate the discussion so that it moves from the generation of ideas to a realistic solution. I would caution you to avoid being a "helicopter professor," taking the term from the way millennial parents hovered over their children (Fang, 2015, para. 1). Thus, balancing your involvement with student and group autonomy is important.

have been working as nurses for a while, the need to teach group skills may be less important than being respectful of each student's need to balance school and other responsibilities. Group projects that require a product have the added element of organization over time zones, which can be an unwelcome stressor for students. For that reason, I would recommend that group projects be kept to a minimum, if required at all.

ADDITIONAL WAYS TO ASSESS AND TEACH

Quizzes

Weekly or module-based quizzes, on the other hand, are used for formative assessment in the online environment, take advantage of the testing effect (Chapter 1), and have many other benefits for students, including improved long-term learning and transfer (Roediger & Karpicke, 2006). Faculty benefit as well because once quizzes are set up, the LMS software will manage them, requiring little faculty monitoring. Although initially writing the questions is time consuming, they can be used for multiple semesters with minimal updating, depending on how often the content changes and the item analyses of the questions. Writing MCQs associated with Bloom's taxonomy is the topic of Chapter 8.

Drill-and-Practice Exercises

Online drill-and-practice exercises that can be set up in the quiz function in any LMS allow students to work through questions on a content area repeatedly until mastery. These exercises can be built into the LMS software and run with little faculty support. Although they require a bit of time to create, they often can be used over and over. Drill-and-practice exercises, from the behaviorist paradigm, are particularly useful for basic skills, such as reading EKGs or x-rays, but can be used to associate research methods with a research question and/or statistical applications.

The Lesson to Encourage If–Then Thinking

Some of the LMSs include software that allow faculty to develop exercises based on if–then thinking. This software in Moodle, called Lesson, can be used in a number of ways. For example, a case study can be created that is followed by MCQs with each question including four options—the right answer and three distractors. Different pathways can be created for each of the four options. Students can head down a plausible, but incorrect, path representing a mistake that is commonly made. They can go so far down the wrong path that the patient's condition deteriorates instead of improving. Students can go through the lesson again and again until they have mastered the case. Multimedia that include video and audio files can be uploaded as part of the case itself or added to one or more of the answers.

PowerPoint is robust software that can be used to create exercises similar to the Lesson in Moodle. Multiple pathways can be created using the hyperlink function to move through the slides in other than a linear fashion. To give you an idea of how this works, think about the game of Jeopardy. Clicking on a square in the game board reveals an answer. Once the player mentally decides what the right question is, he or she clicks on a link to reveal it. A button on that screen routes the player back to the game board. These slides are not in sequential order, thus the game must be run in slide-show mode. This type of game in PowerPoint cannot be used with a group unless group members are all in the same room. However, it is an engaging form of drill and practice that an individual can use to learn content.

Spaced Educational Strategies

Spaced education takes advantage of both the spacing effect, or study that is spaced over a period of time as opposed to massed study or cramming, and the testing effect, the proven finding that frequent testing improves retrieval of memories, retards forgetting, and promotes long-term learning and transfer (Kerfoot et al., 2010; Roediger & Karpicke, 2006; Roediger & Pyc, 2012). Research has shown that frequent testing is more beneficial than repeatedly studying the same material (Roediger & Karpicke, 2006). One means of spacing education is to deliver daily MCQs via e-mail to students containing a link for them to respond within the LMS (Kerfoot et al., 2012). After the student has submitted an answer, he or she is able to see the correct answer and the distractors with rationales as to why they are correct or incorrect. Remedial content is either provided or linked to in order for the student to complete additional study, if necessary. These questions are randomly sent to the student over a specific number of weeks. Using the quiz function of the LMS, a version of this type of study could be set up.

STRATEGIES TO OFFLOAD WORKLOAD

Online courses can take advantage of various strategies to decrease workload without negatively impacting students' learning and achievement of the objectives. As a basis for this discussion, let me address faculty comments listed in the Workload Issues section found in Chapter 3 that indicated to me a lack of understanding in online pedagogy.

Feedback

Replying to every student's post has negative consequences for group discourse and interferes with the development of a community of inquiry (Chapter 10). If faculty post too often, the student-to-student conversation may end and, instead, the focus may shift to student-to-faculty conversation. And, in some instances, students will simply defer to the expert and stop posting.

Feedback to students on assignments does not necessarily need to be text based. Feedback can be provided in a podcast, which is an audio recording in MP3-file format. Most computers have a built-in microphone and recording software that will easily record a podcast. Podcasts can be created on the Mac using GarageBand, a software application that comes with the hardware, or the QuickTime player on the Mac or PC. Another option, called Audacity, is a free download for both operating systems that is very easy to use to create audio files. Students seem to enjoy a reprieve from reading the written word and find feedback in an audio recording useful.

What About Lectures?

Lengthy lectures are not often used in online teaching. Students find mini-lectures of complex material helpful, but these should be limited to 10 to 15 minutes. Podcasts are easy to create and students feel as if they are having a conversation with you about a topic. In addition, students can download an MP3 file to their handheld device and listen while on the go—an appealing quality to the multitasking millennials (Wilson & Gerber, 2008). A podcast can also be created to accompany a slide presentation, in which case students should be directed to open the PowerPoint before starting the audio recording. PowerPoint lectures can also be converted to YouTube videos using screen capture software that is relatively inexpensive. YouTube videos can be downloaded to various handheld devices, providing additional flexibility for study.

Grading Written Assignments

Daggett (2008) has found a unique way to simplify grading on written assignments by compiling a list of frequent comments she finds herself making while grading papers into what she refers to as a *rubric*. This rubric is returned to students with their assignment. Instead of rewriting these comments out each time a mistake is found, she simply writes the code from the rubric that is associated with the error. For example, F6 is a formatting error having to do with quotations. P1 is a punctuation error regarding comma use in a series, and so on. The author notes that this approach has saved many hours of grading and results in a faster turn-around in getting papers back to students.

It is my hope that as you read through this book you will pick up additional tips to help decrease your workload simply by learning more about efficiencies when teaching online and using online pedagogy. Additional strategies, such as peer critique, drill-and-practice exercises, adaptive assessments, and SpacedEd, can be employed as creative teaching strategies that do not involve grading.

Peer Critique

Individual assignments lend themselves nicely to peer critique. This method involves pairing students to provide feedback on each other's work following specific guidelines you have developed. Having guidelines is the key. If students' feedback is not structured, it often will revolve around kudos—how much they liked what the other student did, but providing little actual constructive feedback. The guidelines that you develop should reflect what you would be looking for when grading students' work. This can be accomplished by first making a bulleted list of areas of content you would be looking for when grading. Then, ask specific questions about each area that reflect your metacognitive thinking—the questions you would ask yourself to determine if the student had met the criteria. For example, in the Online Methodologies course I taught, students designed and built their own course in a Moodle shell. Part of the content taught during the semester was interface design, syllabus development, and how to write engaging DQs. The peer critique involved students assessing each of these areas. In terms of interface design, students were asked to comment on the appropriateness of size and type of font, font color selection, organization of the All Weeks section with content not related to a specific week, and the organization of content for weeks 1 and 2. However, the wording of the questions was more general, such as was the organization of week 1 and week 2 similar for intuitive navigation? Is the overall look and feel of the course noncluttered, easy to read, and professional in appearance? Students were asked to provide a rationale for their responses so the student whose course they were reviewing had substantive feedback. Students received two grades for this activity; one providing feedback to a classmate and the other from me based on their Moodle build based on the same requirements.

Peer critique is an excellent way to promote deep learning, as students must apply what they have learned to provide meaningful feedback. In addition, the ability to objectively critique others is a beneficial skill for students to have. Finding the words to praise or criticize without sounding harsh can be difficult. Finding the right word is more easily accomplished in the online environment because students have time to reflect.

Peer critique can save you a great deal of time, as essentially your work has been done for you. The key to successfully using peer critique as an assignment is to provide very specific directions and to use the same criteria when grading both aspects of the assignment—students' critique of a classmate and your assessment of the assignment itself, in the case the Moodle build.

THE TAKE-AWAY

The call to transform nursing education focuses on changing the way we teach and assess nursing students at all educational levels. When considering online education, teaching and assessing are, for the most part, not separate activities, but one in the same. Implementing this concept requires nurse educators to change the way they view formative and summative assessments to take advantage of their teaching value. With discussion boards as the main teaching space in many online courses, the various forms of discussions associated with deliverables may be sufficient to assess the objectives. To avoid busywork for students and faculty, this idea should be carefully considered.

REFERENCES

Baker, D. L. (2011). Designing and orchestrating online discussions. *MERLOT Journal of Online Learning and Teaching, 7*(3), 401–411.

Barrows, H., & Kelson, A. (1996). *Designing a PBL problem.* Unpublished manuscript.

Beattie, V., Collins, B., & McInnes, B. (1997). Deep and surface learning: A simple or simplistic dichotomy? *Accounting Education, 6*(1), 1–12.

Benner, P., Sutphen, M., Leonard, V., & Day, L. (1984/2010). *Educating nurses: A call for radical transformation.* San Francisco, CA: Jossey-Bass.

Brown, J. S., Collins, A., & Duguid, P. (1989). Situated cognition and the culture of learning. *Educational Researcher, 18*(1), 32–42.

Daggett, L. M. (2008). A rubric for grading or editing student papers. *Nurse Educator, 33*(2), 55–56.

Gurrie, C. (2015). Group work: A Millennial myth—Improving group work in the basic course and beyond. *International Journal of Social Science and Humanity, 5*(11), 962–965.

Herrington, J., Reeves, T. C., & Oliver, R. (2010). *A guide to authentic e-learning.* New York, NY: Routledge.

Howe, N., & Strauss, W. (2000). *Millennials rising.* New York, NY: Vintage Books.

Kerfoot, B. P., Baker, H., Pangaro, L., Agarwal, K., Taffet, G., Mechaber, A. J., & Armstrong, E. G. (2012). An online spaced-education game to teach and assess medical students: A multi-institutional prospective trial B. *Academic Medicine, 87*(10), 1443–1449.

Kerfoot, B. P., Fu, Y., Baker, H., Connelly, D., Ritchey, M. L., & Genega, E. M. (2010). Online spaced education generates transfer and improves long-term retention of diagnostic skills: A randomized controlled trial. *Journal of the American College of Surgeons, 211*(3), 331–337.

Koh, H. L., Herring, S. C., & Hew, K. F. (2010). Project-based learning and student knowledge construction during asynchronous online discussion. *Internet and Higher Education, 13,* 284–291.

Lave, J., & Wenger, E. (1991). *Situated learning: Legitimate peripheral participation.* New York, NY: Cambridge University Press.

Leppa, C. J. (2004). Assessing student critical thinking through online discussions. *Nurse Educator, 29*(4), 156–160.

Miller, M. D. (2014). *Minds online: Teaching effectively with technology.* Cambridge, MA: Harvard University Press.

Misanchuk, M., & Anderson, T. (2001, April). Building community in an online learning environment: Communication, cooperation and collaboration. *Proceedings of the Annual Mid-South Instructional Technology Conference,* Murfreesboro, TN. Retrieved from http://files.eric.ed.gov/fulltext/ED463725.pdf

Morgan, K., Williams, K. C., Cameron, B. A., & Wade, C. E. (2014). Faculty perceptions of online group work. *Quarterly Review of Distance Education, 15*(4), 37–41.

Norman, G. R., & Schmidt, H. G. (1992). The psychological basis of problem-based learning: A review of the evidence. *Academic Medicine, 67*(9), 557–565.

Palloff, R. M., & Pratt, K. (2003). *The virtual student: A profile and guide to working with online learners.* San Francisco, CA: Jossey-Bass.

Pintrich, P. R. (2002). The role of metacognitive knowledge in learning, teaching and assessing. *Theory Into Practice, 41*(4), 219–225.

Roediger, H. L., & Karpicke, J. D. (2006). The power of testing memory: Basic research and implications for educational practice. *Perspectives on Psychological Science, 1*(3), 181–210.

Roediger, H. L., & Pyc, M. A. (2012). Applying cognitive psychology to education: Complexities and prospects. *Journal of Applied Research in Memory and Cognition, 1,* 263–265.

Ross, B. (1997). Towards a framework for problem-based curricula. In D. Boud & G. Feletti (Eds.), *The challenge of problem-based learning,* (pp. 28–35). New York, NY: Kogan Page. Retrieved from https://books.google.com/books?id=zvyBq6 k6tWUC&q=ross#v=snippet&q=ross&f=false

Rovai, A. P. (2003, Fall). Strategies for grading online discussions: Effects on discussions and classroom community in Internet-based university courses. *Journal of Computing in Higher Education, 15*(1), 89–107.

Rovai, A. P. (2007). Facilitating online discussions effectively. *Internet and Higher Education, 10,* 77–88.

Schön, D. (1983). *The reflective practitioner.* San Francisco, CA: Jossey-Bass.

Walker, J. T., Martin, T., White, J., Elliott, R., Norwood, A., Mangum, C., & Haynie, L. (2006). Generational (age) differences in nursing students' preferences for teaching methods. *Journal of Nursing Education, 45*(9), 371–374.

Wiggins, G., & McTighe, J. (2005). *Understanding by design* (2nd ed.). Alexandria, VA: Association for Supervision and Curriculum Development.

Wilson, M., & Gerber, L. E. (2008). How generational theory can improve teaching: Strategies for working with the "Millennials." *Currents in Teaching and Learning, 1*(1), 29–44.

Wu, S. Y., Hou, H. T., Hwang, W. Y., & Liu, E. Z. F. (2013). Analysis of learning behavior in problem-solving-based and project-based discussion activities within the seamless online learning integrated discussion (SOLID) system. *Journal of Educational Computing Research, 49*(1), 61–82.

6

Case-Based Authentic
Teaching and Assessment

CONSTRUCTIVISM AND ANDRAGOGY

Constructivism, "a philosophy that people construct their own knowledge through interactions with the environment" (Rovai, 2004, p. 80), is the current instructional philosophy that aligns with the tenets of andragogy. Adult learning theory posits that adults are (a) intrinsically motivated and able to self-direct learning, identify learning needs, and resources; (b) utilize accumulated prior knowledge and experience to direct learning to benefit their future role; and (c) prefer learning to be problem-centered for direct application (Merriam, 2001). Grabinger and Dunlap (1995) operationalized constructivist principles for teaching that incorporate adult learning theory. These principles are as follows:

- *Student responsibility and initiative:* Students are responsible for their learning and are able to self-regulate, which involves reflection on learning.
- *Authentic learning contexts:* Authentic is defined as "realistic and faithful to the original phenomena" (p. 227), indicating that learning should occur within a context relevant to the student's future role.
- *Cooperative support:* Learning within a supportive group teaches group processes, the respect for diverse opinions, brings to light faulty reasoning, and supports coconstruction of knowledge.
- *Generative learning strategies:* Active learning leads to the generation of a product, such as a solution to a problem or assignment.
- *Authentic assessment:* As assessment drives learning, learning should be contextualized and assessed from that context.

Traditional teaching methods, such as the lecture, cannot meet these requirements, but case-based teaching can. McCracken (2015) very aptly describes the case method as one that "combines the power of storytelling with critical discussion, shared experiences, and rigorous academic practice and theory . . . [that] enables the application and testing of theory, it encourages questioning of accepted practice, and it incubates essential dialogue between business practitioners and academics" (p. viii).

Value and Scope of Case-Based Teaching

Various approaches to case-based learning can be used, which range from providing a great deal of information for students to analyze to just a sentence or two indicating an issue that requires the process of inquiry to work through the problem. Which method is chosen depends upon the desired learning outcomes. What differentiates case-based learning from other formats in which readings are assigned followed by lectures and perhaps a test of some sort, is that case-based learning begins with a problem, mimics what the students might encounter in their desired roles, and lacks a road map toward resolution. Overall, cases have the potential to promote "(a) structuring of knowledge for use in clinical contexts; (b) developing of an effective clinical reasoning process; (c) development of effective self-directed learning skills; and (d) increased motivation for learning" (Barrows, 1986, pp. 481–482).

These outcomes are obviously clinically based. However, learning from cases can occur in any course, regardless of the content to be learned. The only limiting factor is faculty's creativity when writing the cases. It is important to note that how faculty manage case-based teaching can make or break the process (discussed in Chapter 11). Case-based teaching must be student directed and not faculty directed; lengthy lectures have no place in case-based learning. If students are guided in identifying their specific learning issues, foundational knowledge and understandings will come to light when they conduct independent study. Also, assessment drives learning, so it is essential that what is assessed "must challenge problem-solving, clinical reasoning and self-directed learning and not primarily emphasize the recall and recognition of facts" (Frederiksen, 1984, as cited in Barrows, 1986, p. 485). This can be accomplished in online case-based teaching because online cases allow for both formative and summative feedback, and can double as teaching methods. In the process of discussing complex cases, students not only learn the content, but also use higher cognitive functions to think critically, which becomes evident from what they post.

Many types of case-based learning are available, but those particularly attuned to an online constructivist model include unfolding cases and problem-based learning (PBL). Before discussing how they differ, let us first look at the process for creating them, the 3C3R method, and what they have in common.

THE 3C3R MODEL

Hung (2009) developed a content and process model for case or problem design for PBL termed *3C3R*. The three Cs represent *content, context,* and *connections* and are the focus of learning in PBL. The three Rs direct cognitive processing and include *researching, reasoning,* and *reflecting.* Incorporating these six variables when writing cases is discussed in detail in the sections that follow.

The Core Components: The Three Cs

Content (Foreground Content)

Two types of information should be included in each case—foreground content and background information that creates context. Foreground content relates directly to the *main* problem to be solved in the case, represents core domain knowledge to be learned, and provides the trigger that will lead to learning in greater depth (Hung, 2009). Because the learners will entertain multiple hypotheses when working through the problem, the case must be designed so that the foreground problem comes to light as one potential hypothesis. However, in the process of researching the problem, students will encounter other potential causes or explanations, which Hung (2009) terms *peripheral domain content,* that create alternative pathways. If developing illness scripts is part of the course design and multiple cases are run simultaneously in different groups, each pathway must lead to a unique, yet plausible, diagnosis. This approach is explained in detail later in this chapter under the Illness Script Assignment section.

Barrows and Kelson (1996) differentiated between a *problem* and an *instance of a problem.* As an example, let us suppose your goal is for students to learn the differential diagnosis of ear pain in the adult, a problem most nurse practitioners (NPs) will encounter in clinical practice. Asking the question, "What causes ear pain in the adult?," will result in all students posting the same information after consulting their textbooks. This is not an *authentic* problem. What is necessary is identifying an *instance* of this problem or specific issue that will occur in real life.

Several instances of ear pain can be introduced by the same brief chief complaint. Let us look at an example. Judy is a 22-year-old otherwise healthy woman who comes into your office complaining of right ear pain for the past 2 days. This complaint of ear pain occurs commonly in primary care practice, meets the definition of authentic, and will engage students as they think like an NP to discover its root cause. Potential causes for this problem include otitis externa, Eustachian tube dysfunction, serous otitis, and otitis media.

For the purpose of illustration, suppose there are four discussion groups responding to this brief chief complaint. If the solution to one case is otitis externa, students will encounter this pathology in addition to other potential diagnoses when researching ear pain, some likely and others less likely for a 22-year-old woman. Those other potential diagnoses are considered peripheral domain content (Hung, 2009) that students will learn about to some degree, but not in as much depth as the one potential hypothesis they will research. Once students review additional pertinent information found in the history, such as a history of recent swimming in a river and findings on the physical exam of a swollen left ear canal limiting view of the tympanic membrane, which appears normal from what can be visualized, they will lean toward a diagnosis of otitis externa. The other three groups will have a similar experience with different information on the history and physical exam (H&P), leading them down different paths in the direction of the other diagnoses. From this case, four instances based on one chief complaint leading to four different diagnoses will be explored in detail with other less common pathologies perhaps mentioned and discussed along the way.

Context (Background Information)

To make the cases messy and complex as well as create an authentic context, background information is added that may or may not be relevant to the problem at hand, yet helps to paint a real-life picture of the complexities of nursing practice. Background information may include socioeconomic status, secondary diagnoses (comorbidities), social issues such as alcohol or drug abuse or a history of smoking, and a complex family history. What this information does is make the patient seem real, adding depth to the case. Although not the main focus or learning outcome of the case, students will be expected to distinguish relevant from irrelevant background information, recognize the significance or salience of the information, and determine whether that data have an impact on the problem, the plan to address the problem, or the patient's general well-being. For example, if the 22-year-old woman with ear pain also had a diagnosis of type 2 diabetes, and her blood sugars have been off baseline since shortly after the pain started, students must now address two issues. This additional data provides an opportunity for students to engage in holistic nursing practice. For nonclinical cases, the same purpose for background information holds true. Think of it as adding a creative touch to the cases to make them seem life-like and real for the student.

Professional Context

In addition, an authentic setting or context must be chosen in which the problem will reveal itself. Along with the background information for the case, the professional context sets the stage for the role students will take in solving the problem. An appropriate context or setting for the RN to bachelor of science in nursing (BSN) student might be within the acute care hospital setting or home health. For the nurse practitioner regardless of population focus, the context would most likely be a primary care setting and for the acute care NP, the setting is likely the hospital.

On the other hand, the professional context may be course-dependent. For example, in a policy course, the setting might be in a meeting room at the local nurses' association headquarters where the student is part of a lobbyist group. Professional context is an important component of authentic cases and assists students with formation into the role they aspire to (Benner, Sutphen, Leonard, & Day, 1984/2010). Because it is role-driven, the professional context may be the same for all cases in a course or program.

Connections

The notion of connections is the final C in the 3C model. Connections made in the profession are difficult to articulate, as they are somewhat intuitive for nurses with experience. They arise out of domain knowledge from the basic sciences, the humanities, and upper division nursing courses, combined with multiple ways of thinking that include critical thinking and diagnostic reasoning. Because our students are RNs with known domain knowledge and varied clinical nursing experience, they will have some understanding of these connections. For example, from a complete history and physical exam of an obese 40-year-old male patient complaining of chest pain, most nurses will pick out potential health risks if additional information is provided that the man smokes two packs of cigarettes per day and lost his father as the result of a myocardial infarction at age 45. From the faculty perspective when writing cases, it is useful to think about past experiences with patient variables and specific diagnoses that students will likely encounter in practice. Including these variables in cases creates a rich, complex, believable context that represents the complexities that can occur in actual nursing practice and gives students the opportunity to connect the dots of provided data to arrive at the best solution given the situation.

The Processing Component: The Three Rs

Researching

Once the problem has been encountered, the next step is research to obtain needed information to solve the problem (Hung, 2006). However, in order to approach the search for information strategically, the problem and goal or end-point must be clearly understood. In terms of a discussion question that may include relevant and irrelevant information by design so that students will gain practice in extracting the salient information from a situation, the problem itself must be clear in their minds. The plan to address or resolve the problem is the goal of an authentic discussion.

Context can influence research by providing a frame of reference that, by default, directs their problem-solving processes. Nursing is a broad field and nurses wear many hats. Context determines the hat the student will wear and the appropriate ways of thinking and methods of researching that go along with that hat.

Reasoning

Because we have not as yet agreed on a term broad enough to encompass critical thinking, diagnostic reasoning, clinical reasoning, or the multiple ways of thinking that nurses must employ, I think about the process of reasoning as "wrestling" with information to arrive at an understanding, as this seems to describe the complex, multifaceted cognitive effort required. Hung (2006) describes the steps of this process, which are:

- Analyzing the nature of all the variables and the interrelationships among them
- Linking newly acquired knowledge with existing knowledge and restructuring their domain knowledge base
- Reasoning causally to understand the intercausal relationships among the variables and the underlying mechanisms
- Reasoning logically to generate and test hypotheses
- Identifying possible solutions and/or eliminating implausible solutions (p. 64)

Reasoning is an iterative process that occurs during and after the process of researching. Thus, these two processes occur simultaneously.

Reflecting

Incorporating reflection as part of a case-based discussion will help students to develop metacognitive strategies. Hung (2006) suggested this occur as both formative and summative processes, a different conceptualization of Schön's (1987) reflection-*in*-action and reflection-*on*-action. Formative reflection or reflection-in-action cannot be separated from researching and reasoning. To some degree, metacognition will guide reasoning.

On the other hand, summative reflection or reflection-on-action occurs at the end of the case and should be a faculty-guided activity, otherwise students may not take time to do it. Asking students to reflect on their research methods, resources used, what they did well, and what they could have done better will promote self-directed learning. Reflecting on the knowledge gained from the case, the reasoning strategies they employed, and what was learned from others in the process of the discussion will help to improve their problem-solving skills (Hung, 2006).

TYPES OF CASE-BASED TEACHING METHODS

Unfolding Cases

Unfolding cases are well named in that the data about the case are given to students in stages, unfolding much like a real-life case in nursing practice in which all pertinent information is not available at the outset, changes with time, or new data are discovered. Each stage may require a shift in thinking and a need to reflect and reevaluate assumptions. These types of cases are well suited to the online environment and are very similar to PBL. How the case unfolds depends on the content, the time element for discussions, the desired learning outcomes, and whether resolution occurs within the discussion or the discussion ends prior to that stage so that students can turn in an individual assignment. For a case in a clinical course with the outcome being a plan of care developed during the discussion, the sequence is shown in Exhibit 6.1. For a nonclinical course, Exhibit 6.2 demonstrates the sequence of unfolding events that might occur.

Each step of the case may span from 2 to 4 days, depending on the requirements of the step and the overall time allotted to the discussion. However, not all steps need be the same number of days. Allotted time must be adequate in order for students to complete their research, synthesize what they have learned, and compose a post. The beauty of this type of unfolding case is that the information provided to students in all steps can be prepared ahead of time. The list of questions provided in Step 2 will not be in response to the actual questions students asked, but instead what faculty deem *should have been asked*. The same is true for findings on the physical exam in Step 3. For Step 4, faculty will need to respond within the discussion to the final plan. Basically, this type of case study will run itself with faculty monitoring students' posts to be sure they do not wander off track, have questions that no one in the group can answer, and

EXHIBIT 6.1
Unfolding Case Format for a Clinical Case

Steps	Information Given to Students	Questions Students Are Asked
1	The patient's problem in the form of a chief complaint is briefly outlined, including the context	1. What is your initial impression of the problem? 2. What are potential explanations for the problem (diagnoses)? 3. What specific questions will you ask the patient (history)?
2	1. Answers to questions students should have asked are given in order to provide the necessary information for students to move on to the next step.	After reviewing answers to the questions, students are asked: 1. Reflect on the questions you asked and those you should have asked based on the information provided. This is a learning activity for you. No need to post what you learned. 2. Are there any changes in your initial impression based on new information provided in the history? 3. How does this new information impact ruling-in or ruling-out your initial diagnosis? 4. Based on the information in the history, what areas will you focus the physical exam on?
3	Findings on the physical exam	1. Are there any changes in your initial impression (diagnosis)? Include rationales as to why. 2. What is your final diagnosis (or differential diagnosis) based on available data?
4	Final diagnosis with rationales related to findings on the history and exam	What is your plan? Include evidence-based rationales for treatment (where available)

meet the learning outcomes. In most learning management systems (LMSs), the documents for Steps 2 and 3 can be set to upload on a certain date and at a certain time, freeing faculty from meeting a midnight deadline, for example.

The downside of this type of unfolding case is that students must post within the time frame for each step. If they do not, they must suffer the consequence of losing points for that step, as once the information has been posted for the next step, the student will have an unfair advantage in constructing his or her post. If this is made clear to students at the outset of the case, they should be able to arrange their time to post in each step in a timely manner.

EXHIBIT 6.2
Unfolding Case Format for a Nonclinical Problem

Steps	Information Given to Students	Questions Students Are Asked
1	A picture of the problem, issue, or dilemma is painted that includes context (background information)	1. What is the problem? Initial description in their own words. 2. What areas of inquiry need to be pursued? 3. Are there any additional questions to be asked or information to be gathered? 4. Who are the stakeholders?
2	Additional information is provided in a narrative format that describes what was learned from inquiry and research Stakeholders are identified and their perspectives stated	1. How has the information provided changed your initial impression of the problem? 2. What additional inquiry is needed? 3. Any additional stakeholders who should be involved? 4. What is your potential solution?
3	The case can unfold in as many steps as necessary to provide twists and turns, giving students additional data to consider	Repeat Steps 1 and 2 until enough information is provided/unveiled for students to come to a conclusion and plan. This will be limited by the allotted time for the discussion.

Problem-Based Learning

PBL is the most researched case-based teaching method to date (Albanese & Mitchell, 1993; Dochy, Segers, Van den Bossche, & Gijbels, 2003; Gijbels, Dochy, Van den Bossche, & Segers, 2005; Shin & Kim, 2013; Vernon & Blake, 1993). However, as Barrows (1986) noted, PBL is "a genus for which there are many species and subspecies" (p. 485). PBL, as described and employed by Barrows and his group at Southern Illinois University's medical school, is considered authentic PBL from which modifications have been made over the years by others, serving to confound research efforts to determine the teaching method's validity (Hung, 2011). In an effort to bring this issue to light and define the various types of PBL, a taxonomy was developed (Barrows, 1986), as was a continuum to create some order (Harden & Davis, 1998), and a framework for analysis of the variations of PBL (Charlin, Mann, & Hansen, 1998). Regardless of the version of case-based teaching employed, writing cases that meet the goals of PBL as originally outlined by Barrows (1986) are listed in the section Tips for Identifying Appropriate Problems for Study later in this chapter.

The PBL process, which was originally carried out in small groups of students who met face to face, will further the understanding of teaching with cases in general, as it is the prototype of case-based teaching (Barrows & Tamblyn, 1980). The steps of the PBL process are as follows:

1. An authentic problem is presented to students without any prerequisite study, that is, reading assignments.
2. Individually, each student reflects on the problem and discusses his or her thoughts with the group so that they may be challenged and evaluated. The scribe takes notes on a whiteboard, listing them in four columns: hypotheses, information synthesis of what is known, learning issues, and action plan.
3. Next, learning issues are identified and assigned to individual students for independent study. Potential resources are identified.
4. When the group reconvenes, each student discusses findings from his or her independent study and relates them back to the problem to evaluate the fit. Hypotheses are revised, new learning issues are identified, and additional information and actions needed are determined. Specific information from the casebook that contains the particulars of the entire case can be requested.

The result of this process is learning from individual study and group work that is then summarized and becomes integrated with the student's prior knowledge and skills. This process may go through several iterations of identifying learning issues, researching them, and reporting on the results to the group before potential solutions are identified.

The PBL process is *facilitated* by a faculty member, called a *tutor*, who asks probing questions without assuming the role of a teacher (i.e., lecturer) and prevents students from researching unfruitful issues. Two additional final steps are valuable for learning that include students reflecting on their reasoning process, providing rationales for their choices, and completing a product, such as a clinical note or other authentic deliverable dictated by the problem.

Online PBL follows much the same process and is quite suited to nursing education for RN–BSN or graduate nursing student for several reasons. Our students' educational backgrounds are quite similar, in that all have completed a basic nursing program and have similar foundational knowledge. Thus, case-based teaching should not be as much of a stretch for our students as for medical students, for example, who come from heterogeneous educational backgrounds. Our students have enrolled in a program because they have a goal or desire to change roles—they want to learn. They are intrinsically motivated, for the most part, and understand being responsible for their learning. They have some measure of clinical experience, have used clinical and diagnostic reasoning, and know what it takes to think like a nurse. They have knowledge, skills, and attitudes on which to build.

However, Barrows (2002) was skeptical that distributed PBL (dPBL) was a realistic expectation, finding online LMSs "cumbersome" (p. 120). However, after completing the PBL tutor training at Southern Illinois University's medical school, visions of creating online PBL flashed through my mind. I knew it could be done. The process is a bit different because students readily identify learning issues and research them independently without being assigned to do so. Also, the casebook is provided. Because of these changes, the process becomes somewhat truncated. Nevertheless, dPBL or online PBL adhere to the original intent and learning outcomes of PBL, especially for the groups of nursing students taking online courses.

Online PBL Process

The online PBL cases unfold in a similar fashion to what occurs in the face-to-face version and mimics how problems evolve in real life, adding to the realism. The path is uncovered as nurses ask questions, analyze data, and use multiple ways of thinking. For clinical cases for NP students, the steps are listed in Box 6.1. The major difference between classroom-based and

---

BOX 6.1
STEPS OF ONLINE PROBLEM-BASED LEARNING PROCESS

1. *Encounter a problem* in the form of brief demographic information such as gender and age of the patient and a chief complaint (Day 1–2).
2. *Hypothesis generation:* Each student develops a prioritized list of differential diagnoses, posts them, and states which one he or she plans to explore in more depth. Each student's next post on the chosen potential diagnosis will include associated pathophysiology, epidemiology, additional expected signs and symptoms if any, and a rationale as to why the student feels this diagnosis could explain the chief complaint (Days 3–5).
3. *Data provided:* Faculty then provide a complete history and physical exam (H&P) on the patient containing both relevant and irrelevant information. After reviewing the H&P, the student's next post will include his or her thoughts on how the data support ruling in or ruling out the chosen potential diagnosis. As students post, each will also comment on his or her colleague's thoughts, often in a debate-style dialogue until a final diagnosis (or list of differential diagnoses) is reached (Days 6–8).
4. *Plan of care:* Two choices exist for continuing the case. Discussion can continue as students collaborate to develop a plan of care for the patient and are graded on their individual contributions to the plan (Days 9–12). Or the discussion can end with each student writing a plan of care as an individual assignment. The due date for this assignment can be assigned outside of the 2-week interval for each case.

online PBL is the step of identifying potential hypotheses for the chief complaint and learning issues. Students post their list of potential hypotheses, identify the one they will work on, and begin independent research. Faculty should be vigilant during this step to avoid problems. If two students indicate in separate posts that they plan to work on the same potential hypothesis, an e-mail to both students is necessary to communicate which student should proceed and which should choose another topic, so no confusion occurs. In the process of that research, they will identify areas that they do not understand. These will become their own personal learning issues that they will continue to look into until they reach understanding or post an inquiry to the group. Alternatively, after posting their initial perspectives, feedback may be forthcoming from other students and faculty to help the student connect the dots.

Both unfolding cases and PBL are engaging ways for students to learn in online group discussions that give them the opportunity to test their wings thinking like an NP, researcher, administrator, or educator. The process provides vicarious experience in managing complex patients with feedback from faculty along the way. Working in a small group, students can make their thoughts public, view the perspectives of others, receive feedback from faculty and peers, reflect on their position, and revise if needed.

CASE DEVELOPMENT PROCESS

Logistical Issues to Consider

Multiple logistical issues similar to those encountered with discussion questions, which are discussed in Chapter 5 (Precursors to Successful Discussions section), should be addressed up front. Additional logistical issues specific to case-based teaching include the organization of cases throughout multiple courses, the number of cases to be discussed in the course, and the number of discussion groups.

Organization of Cases

The first decision to be made is whether the content will be spread out over several semesters or taught in one course only. This is especially relevant to clinically oriented courses. If the content is to be spread over two or more courses, for example, the best approach is to let common chief complaints guide the process and not body systems, acute or chronic health issues, or other demographic identifiers such as the patient's age. Students will encounter problems identified by the chief complaint and/or signs and symptoms for NP students. When I was practicing as an NP, I thought of it as *What is behind door number one?*, indicating the broad and unpredictable nature of primary care practice. However, the other impetus for organizing cases by chief complaint is to compare and contrast the aspects on the history and exam that result in varied diagnoses.

If content is to be spread out over two or more courses, I recommend creating a course content map discussed later in the chapter (see Mapping of Outcomes and Content, Course Content Map) that indicates what specific content belongs in each course to ensure that any repetition is done by design and not by poor planning, and that essential content is not overlooked. The course content map is discussed in the section so named later in the chapter.

Number of Cases for the Course

The number of cases to be developed for a specific course is often dictated by the amount and type of content to be addressed. However, this may also hinge on other factors, such as the number of weeks in the semester and the number of students in the course, which is information readily available from administration before the semester starts. Whether each group will discuss the same case or different cases will also impact the number of cases needed for the course. If the plan is for each group to discuss a different instance of the problem (Barrows & Kelson, 1996), which is discussed earlier in the chapter, faculty will need to determine if an adequate number of instances can be identified for each content area to create a case for each discussion group. If not, another option is two or more discussion groups can discuss the same instance. If this occurs, it is important to block each of these groups from seeing other groups' posts while the discussion is in progress, which is a setting in the LMS. Also, if different instances of the same issue are planned, time should be allotted for students to review the other cases, or a quiz developed that will review all instances so that students learn the full scope of that issue. The final logistical issue to consider is whether discussions are the main means of teaching and assessment in the course or if additional teaching methods such as mini-lectures and additional assessments such as quizzes are needed.

Accompanying the various types of case-based learning of which PBL is the prototype, a variety of processes have been developed to create the cases (Azer, Peterson, Guerrero, & Edgren, 2012; Barrows & Kelson, 1996; Barrows & Tamblyn, 1980; Dolmans, Snellen-Balendong, Wolfhagen, & van der Vleuten, 1997; Drummond-Young & Mohide, 2001; Hung, 2006, 2009; Nathanson, 1998; Savin-Baden, 2007). The process I use to develop cases is a combination of these processes, organized using the 3C3R method outlined by Hung (2006).

As an aside, it is important to recognize the differences between the role of an instructional designer and that of the content expert when designing cases. Instructional designers are process experts in that they are adept at directing the process of course content development. Content experts are, just as the name suggests, experts in the area of content of the course being developed. Hung's (2009) perspective is that of an instructional designer. However, his article that outlines the steps of the 3C3R process seems to indicate that the instructional designer can develop the cases. Although it may be possible that an instructional designer also has specific content expertise, this is not a common occurrence in nursing. Content experts with rich clinical experience who have walked the walk and can convert that experience to complex cases are needed for authentic case development.

I recommend using the Backward Design (Wiggins & McTighe, 2005) to begin the process of developing cases. The steps are as follows:

1. *Identify outcomes:* Identify desirable outcomes from the course objectives; content required to pass certification boards (if applicable); and how the knowledge, skills, and attitudes will be used in future practice. The product of this stage is the *course content map,* which contains an outline of foreground content and background information, and is discussed in detail in section Mapping of Outcomes and Content later in this chapter.
2. *Evidence of learning and learning experiences:* Determine what will constitute evidence of learning for each case. As the cases themselves include formative and summative assessments, they may be considered the main means of assessment in the course. In this step you will drill down to the major content that needs to be assessed and use that information to develop a *cognitive case map for each case,* which is discussed in the Cognitive Case Map section later in this chapter. After completing the cognitive case map, you are ready to write the cases.
3. *Additional teaching methods or assessments:* Determine if additional learning experiences are necessary based on the complexity of the content being taught. Decide how that content will be taught at this juncture, such as quizzes, drill-and-practice exercises, and so on.

Two additional steps in the process are to conduct a case review with other faculty and develop the grading rubric(s). A case review allows other faculty teaching the course or colleagues to review the cases to locate any inconsistencies or issues before the cases go to students. This is discussed later in the chapter under Case Review.

It is hoped that examining each step in greater detail will provide the reader with enough information to utilize the process when developing a curriculum or course in which teaching is done online with cases. Doing so will also outline an instructional design process that may seem somewhat foreign to nursing faculty.

STAGES OF CASE DESIGN

Stage 1: Identify Outcomes

The first stage is shared with the Backward Design process of Wiggins and McTighe (2005) and encompasses understanding the outcomes of the course (from the objectives) and how these outcomes mesh with programmatic, credentialing, and accreditation standards. Ideally, this was taken into consideration and incorporated into the course objectives, which were written in broad terms as described in Chapter 4. Course objectives provided by the curriculum committee must be used when determining what is to be learned and assessed in the course. They cannot be altered in any way.

Remember that *all objectives must be assessed*. When objectives are broadly written, a fair amount of academic freedom exists when choosing the teaching strategies and methods of assessment. However, the downside of broadly written objectives is that they lack the detail needed when drilling down to write the cases. Because of this, faculty are often tempted to write subobjectives for each case or module in the course.

Subobjectives for each case can be cumbersome, and I do not recommend this practice for several reasons. First, although the original understanding that short-term memory can hold only seven pieces (plus or minus two) of data is being called into question, the idea that short-term memory is limited persists. With rehearsal, information can make it into long-term memory. However, retrieving it for later use depends on the availability of cues for recall (Miller, 2014). My point in mentioning this is that it is doubtful whether students will expend that much energy with a long list of subobjectives. Second, from the students' perspective, objectives are written to guide learning. When using cases as the foundation for learning, providing too much direction for students could backfire and make them more dependent when your goal is to promote self-directed learning. So, sharing the subobjectives with students would be counterproductive. Third, goals and objectives may not be sufficient to guide teaching. A better approach exists, which is a cognitive case map for each case. This map is a helpful tool for faculty that details the learning outcomes of each case and provides a road map to guide faculty as they facilitate the discussions so that the desired learning occurs and students remain on track. Details on how to develop the cognitive case map are discussed later in this chapter under the section so named.

Stage 2: Determine Evidence of Learning and Plan Learning Experiences

When creating a course for the online environment, Stages 2 and 3 in the original Backward Design process (Wiggins & McTighe, 2005) cannot really be separated. What serves as assessments when teaching face to face, become both assessments and teaching methods in the online environment. However, additional teaching methods might be required. When planning a course, the decision to use assessments that double as teaching methods should be made first before considering additional educational needs.

Keep in mind that authentic cases discussed by small groups of students can serve as formative and summative assessments and the main teaching strategy for the course. Additional methods that serve both teaching and assessment functions, such as multiple-choice quizzes, may be used to augment content being learned in the cases and as practice for certification boards. Most LMS include software that will allow you to create multiple-choice questions (MCQs) and cases using if–then logic that are completely managed by the LMS software and that faculty do not need to monitor.

Case Development

Tips for Identifying Appropriate Problems for Study

Barrows and Kelson (1996) identified characteristics of an authentic case that faculty can use as a guide. They should:

- Be ill structured, messy, and open ended (para. 7)
- Present with insufficient information to solve the problem (para. 8)
- Require that the learner evaluate the reliability and significance of information and resources used to solve the problem (para. 9)
- Often result in decisions being made "in the absence of certainty" (para. 12)
- Challenge the problem solver to "stretch creative thinking" (para. 13)

To this list, Nathanson (1998) added that cases should be user friendly so students do not struggle to understand the case itself or to identify the problem. He also included that cases should be consistent with the course objectives, written in a similar format throughout the course, and challenging to students. Dolmans et al. (1997) recommend that the case should "enhance students interest in the subject matter, by sustaining discussion about possible solutions and facilitating students to explore alternatives" (p. 185). Clearly, these characteristics meet the definition of authentic and ill structured outlined in Chapter 5. They also set the stage for writing cases that mirror the challenges and complexity of daily nursing practice.

Consideration of the level of problem difficulty and the multiple ways of thinking required should be compared to the students' level of prior knowledge. If problem difficulty and reasoning ability are mismatched, students will either be frustrated by a problem that is too difficult or bored by one that is too easy. Consider where the course falls in the program and students' familiarity with and ability to grasp case-based learning, and gage case complexity accordingly. Starting the course with a less complex case may be the best approach.

Engaging cases are a challenge to write if one is accustomed to asking questions requiring fact-based answers. However, past experiences in clinical or other practice areas are often good places to start to create complex cases with inherent problems to solve or issues to address.

Questions to Ask When Beginning to Develop Case Studies

To start the process of actually penning the cases, consider convening a group of faculty to assist under your direction. When beginning to develop case studies, the questions to ask are included in Box 6.2.

Mapping of Outcomes and Content

Course Content Map

If cases will be used in more than one course, a course content map that indicates what specific content belongs in each course will be very useful,

---

BOX 6.2
QUESTIONS TO ASK WHEN BEGINNING
TO DEVELOP CASE STUDIES

1. What is it about this *content* that students will encounter as problems in their future role? *(Foreground content)*
2. What additional variables are necessary to paint a realistic picture of a complex and messy situation? What other variables (health disparities, ethical issues, etc.) would enhance the case and make it more realistic? *(Background information)*
3. What is the *professional context* in which this problem will reveal itself? Is it an outpatient setting, primary care office, etc.? *(Background information)*

especially if multiple faculty are planning and teaching those courses. An Excel spreadsheet or a table in Word can be used to develop a course content map. Headings on the columns should include:

1. *Foreground content:* The main domain knowledge to be learned and the problem to be addressed.
2. *Background information* that may or may not be relevant to the problem at hand, but that creates an authentic, real-life messy context, adding depth and breadth to the problem.
3. *Professional context:* Include professional context at the top of the case map if it is the same for all cases. If it will differ for each case, create a separate column.

When developing the course content map, I recommend that any abbreviations used in the document be standardized and an index compiled that indicates what each abbreviation means. For example, if these are clinical cases and type 2 diabetes mellitus recurs throughout the case map, either as the foreground problem to be addressed or as background issue or comorbidity, using the abbreviation DM2 to indicate the disease will make searching the document easy to accomplish in order to determine if the content surrounding this common malady is adequately addressed. Similarly, abbreviations for classes of medications can be used instead of the individual brand or generic names to ensure review of those classes of drugs commonly used in practice. A brief excerpt of the course content map is shown in Exhibit 6.3.

Cognitive Case Map

Instead of writing subobjectives for each case that faculty cannot share with students, I have found what Hung (2009) terms a *cognitive map* written for each case to be more useful. I have renamed this map as the cognitive case map in order to distinguish it from the course content map, which contains a summary of foreground content and background information for *all* cases in the course or program.

The cognitive case map is a guide of each case for faculty, which (a) includes the minute details of the content, context, and connections students should explore during the discussion that serves to guide faculty when facilitating discussion groups and scaffolding student learning; (b) serves as a reference for faculty to identify learning outcomes necessary to meet the objectives; (c) provides a road map of content to be learned in order for students to function effectively in practice and to pass certification boards; and (d) becomes the foundation for development of the case-grading rubric. Content areas of the map for each case, shown in Box 6.3, should follow the sections of the case and include the following for each case.

EXHIBIT 6.3
Course Content Map Example

Case Number 1.1	Foreground Content	Background Information			
Chief complaint given to students: *Brittany Chapman is a 20-year-old college student c/o "sore throat"*		Professional context: *University student health*			
Diagnosis for this case: *Strep pharyngitis*					
Diagnoses for other cases: *Mononucleosis, Herpes simplex, Allergies*					
Potential diagnoses: (Peripheral domain content)		Comorbidities	Meds/Allergies	Social History	Family History
GERD Allergies Viral infection Peritonsillar abscess Epiglottitis	Retropharyngeal abscess Herpes simplex Influenza Gonorrhea	Seasonal allergies Acne	Doxycycline 100 mg bid Cetirizine (Zyrtec) 10 mg qd Sulfa—rash	College student, substance abuse; ETOH—three beers/night Smokes when drinks + second-hand smoke elevated BP on exam	Father died of stroke at age 62; history of chronic depression; smoker and alcohol abuse Mother, age 58, obese with HTN and DM2. Mother has remarried. Three siblings: A&W

A&W, alive and well; bid, twice a day; BP, blood pressure; c/o, complaining of; DM2, type 2 diabetes mellitus; ETOH, ethanol; GERD, gastroesophageal reflux disease; HTN, hypertension; qd, every day.

Note: See the Appendix for a blank version of this template.

BOX 6.3
CONTENTS OF COGNITIVE CASE MAP

- The chief complaint or introduction to the case that faculty provide for students
- Hypotheses students should mention and the correct solution(s) for each case
- Specific content to be discussed in each step
- A list of additional background information that students should address
- Supporting documents that students will be given, such as the history and physical exam, diagnostic results, and so on
- A list of up-to-date evidence-based references that students are expected to locate and cite in their postings
- General guidelines for facilitation (see Chapter 11) provided with the first case

---

If for some reason the cases are revised after the first iteration, be sure to update these documents as well. Providing this depth of information for faculty coteaching the course, be they new to teaching online or veterans of the format, will promote consistent responses to students' questions and facilitation of the cases.

The cognitive case map can be created in a table in Word or an Excel spreadsheet. An example of a completed map for the 22-year-old woman with ear pain is shown in Exhibit 6.4.

Additional Assessments and Teaching Strategies

Iterative Grading

Additional authentic *products* of various types of case-based discussions might include an illness script, SOAP (subjective, objective, assessment, and plan) or progress note, a podcast of a case presentation or SBAR (situation, background, assessment, recommendation) report, a note to a senator, or evaluation of a research report, to name a few possibilities. These assignments become teaching tools if they are graded in an *iterative* manner. By this I mean providing formative feedback that does not include faculty's corrections, but instead asks questions to point students toward changes that will help improve their work. The assignment is then returned to students to make the necessary changes before resubmitting. This process may take several iterations, and does increase the workload for faculty. Once the assignment is done well and meets the criteria for full

EXHIBIT 6.4

Cognitive Case Map Example

Case Number 1	Initial Content Provided	Connections
Chief complaint given to students: 22-year-old woman with right ear pain		
Professional context: Primary care private office		
Expected list of potential diagnoses: Otitis media Otitis externa Eustachian tube dysfunction Serous otitis TMJ syndrome Cellulitis Trauma Abscess in ear canal		Students may come up with additional potential diagnoses, but what is listed here should be mentioned
Content Provided as Case Unfolds		
History	Healthy female with seasonal allergies taking cetirizine (Zyrtec) 10 mg qd Just returned from vacation—tubing on Colorado River and fell in several times, hitting right side of head on the inflated raft they were riding in Felt right ear gradually plug up during flight home to New York from Colorado Rates pain as 6 on 1–10 scale Family history—adopted Social history—ETOH—two to four beers/day on regular basis (not just on vacation)	This will narrow potential hypotheses, so students should discuss ones that are less likely based on the history alone. Connections from history: Otitis media Otitis externa—from river water Serous otitis—from Eustachian tube dysfunction due to barotrauma of flying Trauma—from hitting right side of head when fell out of raft Abscess in ear canal—again, from river water

(continued)

145

EXHIBIT 6.4
Cognitive Case Map Example (*continued*)

Case Number 1	Initial Content Provided	Connections
Exam	BP 140/96 P - 76 Ht. 5′5″ Wt. 155 BMI 25.8 Heart, lungs, abdominal exam—normal findings HEENT normal except for right ear canal, which is symmetrically swollen so that TM is only partially visible. What can be seen appears normal. No drainage in canal. Right pinna is minimally swollen without heat or redness. Hearing Weber lateralizes to right ear; AC > BC bilaterally No cervical lymphadenopathy	Possible diagnoses limited, but otitis media cannot be ruled out. Should talk about Weber and Rinne's result, expected for conductive loss, which may be due to canal swelling. BP elevation may be due to pain, but will need follow-up and may be related to BMI. Students should ask about risk factors.
Lab	None to review	
Assessment	Otitis externa Possible otitis media Overweight Elevated BP	
Plan	Antibiotic according to current evidence-based guidelines Acetaminophen for pain Keep ear canal dry Follow-up 5 days or sooner if pain worsens	Plan for follow-up for BP, weight, assess risk factors for HTN, heart disease.

AC, air conduction; BC, bone conduction; BMI, body mass index; BP, blood pressure; ETOH, ethanol; HEENT, head, ears, eyes, nose, and throat; Ht., height; HTN, hypertension; P, pulse; TM, tympanic membrane; TMJ, temporomandibular joint; qd, every day; Wt., weight.

Note: See the Appendix for a blank version of this template.

points, a grade can be assigned. However, if an assignment, such as a SOAP note or SBAR report, is a recurring assignment based on the various cases in the course, using the iterative method of providing feedback will improve students' subsequent performance on each assignment, thus shortening the grading time.

A note of caution is in order when grading using the iterative process. Some students will take advantage of the iterative process and not put forth their best effort when turning in the first iteration. My rule of thumb is that if I find myself working harder than it appears the student is, I end the process, describe what the student could have done to improve the product, and provide a grade based on the rubric for the assignment.

To avoid changing the grading rules midstream, two alternative approaches are useful. In both approaches, I will mention in the description of the assignment that it will be graded on an iterative basis and explain what that means. In one approach, I will limit my involvement to two readings and include this in the instructions. After the first read, I will return it to the student with feedback, assigning a grade after the student has made changes and I have read it the second time. In the other approach, I will grade the first iteration and make a note of it, return the assignment with feedback, and assign a grade for the second iteration. The final grade the student earns for the assignment becomes the average of the grades on the two iterations. This encourages students to do their best on the first iteration.

Illness Script Assignment

Developing and organizing instances of cases by a similar chief complaint that unfolds differently for each group leading to unique diagnoses is a means of promoting clinical reasoning and the development of a mental model called an *illness script*. An illness script is a mental representation of a clinical problem based on a similar organizing feature such as a diagnosis, presenting sign or symptom, or a syndrome that acts as a *trigger* for later retrieval from cognitive structures. Storing cases by this organizing feature helps build complex mental models of the feature (a schema), and promotes storage in cognitive structures as related cases (Bowen, 2006). When this specific trigger is encountered in clinical practice, the clinician retrieves the mental model of a previously stored case to compare it to the one at hand.

From the outcomes perspective, this approach requires careful planning to determine diagnoses, associated chief complaints, and so on, that are commonly seen in clinical practice. At the end of the discussion, students are required to review the other cases they did not actually participate in, comparing and contrasting similar features and identifying the main feature that changed how each case unfolded, such as a finding on the history or exam, pathophysiological insult, or predisposing condition. Once the pivotal feature is identified and associated with the final diagnosis in each case, it becomes the unique feature that differentiates the outcome for each case. Students then realize that this defining feature should be sought out early during the history or exam when encountering that specific chief complaint.

If, for example, four groups of five students were assigned a case in which the chief complaint was of a 22-year-old woman with pain in her left ear, each case would unfold differently leading to the most common causes of ear pain, such as otitis externa, Eustachian tube dysfunction, serous otitis, and otitis media. At the end of the case and after review of the other three cases they did not directly participate in, students will understand the key factor instrumental in changing the course of diagnostic reasoning and, ultimately, the diagnosis. One group may have been given information in the H&P that the woman had just returned from a 3-hour flight while battling an upper respiratory infection, whereas another group learned that she had recently returned from a vacation that included tubing down the Colorado River with several unplanned dunks in the water. Requiring an illness script as a product of the case discussion graded in an iterative fashion will promote the development of a mental model for that chief complaint that includes four potential diagnoses, each associated with a unique trigger leading to each diagnosis. This serves to store a chief complaint in cognitive structures in the same manner in which it will be later retrieved. Such an assignment is called an illness script (see Durham, Fowler, & Kennedy [2014] for more details on this assignment).

To standardize the format of the illness script assignment, a template is provided for students containing the pertinent headings such as working hypothesis, predisposing conditions, pathophysiological insult, discriminating features such as expected findings on the history and exam, and defining feature or qualifier. An example of a completed illness script for the case of the 22-year-old female with ear pain is presented in Exhibit 6.5.

SOAP Note Assignment

The SOAP note or progress note as a product of a case discussion deserves special mention here. The subjective, objective, assessment, and plan framework of a SOAP note has served as the universal format for the note since the 1960s when Dr. Lawrence Weed (Weed, 1968) introduced the problem-oriented medical record (POMR). This organizing framework served to standardize documentation and improve communication among health care providers.

When done well, the SOAP note paints a picture of the patient encounter so that anyone reading it could visualize the actual event and understand what had occurred. Inherent yet not articulated in the note was the diagnostic reasoning process of the writer. Over time, the SOAP note became linked to reimbursement for the visit, with certain content required

EXHIBIT 6.5
Illness Script Example

Case: 22-year-old woman with right ear pain

Working Hypothesis	Predisposing Conditions	Pathophysiological Insult	Discriminating Features (Such as Expected Findings on the History and Exam)	Defining Feature or Qualifier
Otitis externa	Swimming in unclean water Trauma from Q-tip usage	Disruption of normal skin defense mechanisms due to trauma	Painful ear Conductive hearing loss Drainage from ear Swollen ear canal obstructing visualization of TM	Increased pain with movement of pinna or pressure on tragus Symmetrical swelling of ear canal
Otitis media	Due to URI, sinusitis, or allergies	Bacteria, fungus, or virus that disrupts function of the cilia in the Eustachian tube; stagnating fluids	Painful ear Conductive hearing loss TM dull, red with landmarks not visible	Appearance of TM—red, dull
Serous otitis	URI, sinusitis, or resolving acute otitis media Barotrauma	Eustachian tube dysfunction resulting in inability of cilia to move fluid	Fullness and loss of hearing more common complaints than pain Conductive hearing loss	Appearance of TM—yellow in color
Abscess in ear canal	Trauma from Q-tip use	Normal skin defenses lost and infection intervenes	Painful ear Depending on size of swelling, conductive hearing loss may result	Asymmetrical swelling of ear canal. Abscess may be visible.

TM, tympanic membrane; URI, upper respiratory infection.

Note: See the Appendix for a blank version of this template.

in the note to bill at each level (Larimore & Jordan, 1995). This change in focus for the note often resulted in extraneous information being added so that reimbursement was higher for the visit, impacting the note's value as a glimpse into the diagnostic reasoning process of the writer.

With the advent of the electronic medical record (EMR), the intent of documenting the patient encounter shifted further along the continuum from an accurate description of what occurred, the ability to infer the diagnostic reasoning process of the writer, and the result of the visit to what elements were required for greater reimbursement. Some EMRs include a clinical decision support system, prompts, and a series of dropdown menus and check boxes that have changed the cognitive processes required to document a patient encounter from recall to recognition and the process itself from active thinking to passive doing. Although the EMRs may improve clinical performance of practitioners and boost patient safety, the clinical reasoning required in order to write a note has been lost. At least from a practical perspective, the need to teach students the format of the SOAP note, what is included in each step, and how to write a useful note has become obsolete. However, because the SOAP note is an excellent means of observing students' diagnostic reasoning abilities, I feel it still has value as an assignment to follow an online case discussion. What should be included in the note can be reviewed in Box 6.4.

SOAP notes, I believe, continue to hold value as a useful method of teaching, from which students' process of diagnostic reasoning is revealed. Although students' early notes are typically much too lengthy, working with faculty in an iterative process will help them shorten the note, include only essential elements, and make their diagnostic reasoning process obvious. This type of assignment can be the product of a case-based group discussion that ended prior to the assessment and plan phases. It is also an obvious assignment from the clinical setting, especially when students are unable to use the EMR where they are precepting due to administrative decisions. The downside of a SOAP note based on a clinical encounter is that faculty cannot verify the details of the patient encounter or who actually did the diagnostic reasoning—the student or the preceptor.

SBAR or Case Presentation Assignment

The ability to succinctly summarize a patient's condition in the acute care hospital or a patient encounter in the primary care setting is a valuable skill for nurses. The SBAR report is the hand-off that occurs in hospitals at the change of shift or whenever a summary of the patient is needed (Cornell, Gervis, Yates, & Vardaman, 2013). When presenting a case to an NP colleague or physician, NPs do a case presentation, also referred to as a *bullet presentation*, which follows a format similar to SBAR. Other nonclinical applications of verbal reporting might include an elevator speech when

---

BOX 6.4
CONTENT FOR SOAP NOTES

- Subjective
  - The chief complaint (CC)
  - Pertinent positives that serve to further describe the chief complaint from the attributes of a symptom
  - Pertinent negatives that *reflect potential differential diagnoses*[a] (not random symptoms) that the student has ruled out based on the history alone listed as a series of *denies*. Pertinent positive and negative social and family history information should be included here as well.
- Objective
  - Focused physical exam findings that include *only* those that will help rule in or rule out the diagnoses being considered.[a] The exam should validate or refute what was learned from the history.
  - Only pertinent diagnostic and laboratory data that contribute to decision making at the visit[a]
- Assessment
  - The diagnosis or a differential diagnosis[a]
  - What is listed should follow logically from what is included in the subjective and objective portions of the note.
- Plan
  - Diagnostic tests to be done with a specified time frame
  - Medications initiated or discontinued
  - Patient and family education
  - Time frame for follow-up

[a]This limited focus is essential and is what reveals the diagnostic reasoning capability of the writer.

---

preparing those soon to graduate for job interviews, an approach to a busy senator to briefly summarize pending legislation that you want her to support, and a summary of a research proposal to a potential funding source. To help hone students' skills in making these verbal presentations, an assignment that consists of a brief 1- to 2-minute podcast created using the microphone built into most computers can be assigned as an authentic summative assessment. An MP3 file can then be created and uploaded as an assignment. Special accommodation may be required, however, as these files can be too large to upload to the LMS. If faculty provide formative feedback and allow the student to redo the podcast, learning will occur and result in improved performance.

To create authentic assignments that promote skills needed in practice, one need only look to the role and those skills that are most valued. These assignments are challenging for students, yet worth their time and effort.

Quizzes to Support Learning From Cases

To take advantage of the testing effect (Roediger & Karpicke, 2006) that is discussed in Chapter 1 (Testing Effect and Spaced Study section), frequent, low-stakes multiple-choice quizzes can be planned to support learning with cases. Here the purpose is somewhat different in that the quizzes will help students make connections that are essential for practice. They are somewhat of a summary of the learning outcomes of the cases to be sure that students learned what was intended and are able to transfer what was learned. Although these are formative in nature, points are assigned as extrinsic motivation for students to take them seriously. I would recommend allowing two opportunities to take these quizzes, with answers for incorrect responses available 24 hours after the quiz closes. This practice will support long-term retention of the content and avoid the *negative suggestion effect*, which indicates that students may later think an incorrect response was correct (Roediger & Karpicke, 2006).

THOUGHTS ON GRADING CASE-BASED DISCUSSIONS

For case-based discussions, the rubric should follow expectations for posting on the elements listed in the cognitive case map. Specific instructions on how to develop an analytic or grading rubric are discussed in Chapter 9. However, for the clinical case we have been discussing, the suggested performance criteria are listed in Box 6.5.

BOX 6.5
PERFORMANCE CRITERIA FOR GRADING RUBRIC
FOR CLINICAL CASE

- Identification of potential hypotheses
- Elaboration of one hypothesis, including pathophysiology, additional signs and symptoms
- Salient features from the history and physical exam as related to the student's hypothesis and if they help to rule in or rule out that hypothesis
- Final diagnosis or differential diagnoses
- Plan of care that includes the steps
- Timing and number of posts—both initial post for each section (perhaps) and responses to colleagues
- Appropriate references and citation of research explored

CASE REVIEW

Experience has taught me about what Wiggins and McTighe (2005) refer to as the "Expert Blind Spot" (p. 138). This phenomenon occurs when experts have difficulty walking in the shoes of the novice as they create course content that will be new and/or unfamiliar to the novice. The problem manifests itself through steps that are omitted or huge leaps made.

I must share a humorous example of why it is so important to have multiple eyes on each case prior to making them active in a course. When I first became involved in transitioning an NP program from classroom-based to online, I developed an H&P template containing all normal findings. My plan was to change the specific areas in this document to other than normal findings as required by specific cases the team was writing. That seemed to be the most efficient approach, rather than recreating a new H&P for each case. One case we created was of a male with a specific complaint. What we failed to do was change the endocrine/reproductive areas on the H&P, and the faculty member who proofread that document did not catch the error. We were mortified when a student e-mailed to ask why this male patient had female reproductive organs on exam!

Members of the case development team should review all the cases for clarity, typos, and frank content errors. I recommend reading them very slowly and out loud, as if *hearing* them for the first time from the student's perspective. I also recommend using track changes in Word to highlight these changes and review them in a round-robin fashion before being finalized. Because students often focus on inconsistencies and errors that impede continued work on the case, taking the extra time to complete this step is essential.

INSTRUCTIONS FOR STUDENTS

Directions that anticipate what students will need to understand and questions they will ask in order to be successful in a course based on case-based learning should be ready when the course opens. These instructions should include information about self-directed learning in general and how the case-based approach differs from teaching methods they have most likely experienced in other courses or educational programs. Covering these steps is essential and will save time for faculty and decrease anxiety and frustration for students.

I recommend that you take the time to explain, in an announcement in the LMS or as part of a podcast that reviews the syllabus, how the steps of the cases will unfold and the timing for each phase. Although the dates for each discussion are included in the syllabus, dates for the steps will most likely not be, as this would result in a lengthy syllabus. The steps that will remain constant for each case can be outlined in the student instructions in this manner:

1. *Phase 1 starts on Monday at 8:00 a.m., and will end on Friday at 11:55 p.m.*
2. *Phase 2 starts on Friday at 11:55 p.m., and will end on Monday at 8:00 a.m.*
3. *Phase 3 starts on Monday at 8:00 a.m., and will end on Friday at 11:55 p.m.*

As each discussion begins, it is prudent to post an announcement that specifies the exact days and dates for each phase. Also include expectations of timing and number and length of required posts, whether students will be able to see their group-mates' posts before they post for the first time, and the expectations for the quality of references. Although this information is most likely included in the grading rubric or syllabus, students will appreciate having all the instructions in one place. Do tell them where the rubric is posted in the LMS and remind them to review it prior to preparing their posts.

Anticipating student issues and misunderstandings becomes easier each time the course is taught. Overcompensating with instructions at the outset of the course may be the best approach. Other suggestions and tips for course management are presented in Chapter 12.

THE TAKE-AWAY

Teaching with cases is an engaging method that students really seem to embrace if the cases are authentic and mimic the complexities of nursing practice. Students quickly take on the role they aspire to in order to wrestle with the content and multiple ways of thinking. The key for faculty is organizing the cases across the course or multiple courses using the course content map to assure that essential content is discussed, repetition is planned, and both practice and credentialing requirements are considered. Developing a cognitive case map for each case will save time once the course is underway and will ensure that students meet the learning outcomes and you have a road map to guide you as you guide the students.

REFERENCES

Albanese, M. A., & Mitchell, S. (1993). Problem-based learning: A review of literature on its outcomes and implementation issues. *Academic Medicine, 68*(1), 52–81.

Azer, S. A., Peterson, R., Guerrero, A. P. S., & Edgren, G. (2012). Twelve tips for constructing problem-based learning cases. *Medical Teacher, 34,* 361–367.

Barrows, H. (2002). Is it truly possible to have such a thing as dPBL? *Distance Education, 23*(1), 119–122.

Barrows, H., & Kelson, A. (1996). *Designing a PBL problem*. Unpublished manuscript.

Barrows, H. S. (1986). A taxonomy of problem-based learning methods. *Medical Education, 20*, 481–486.

Barrows, H. S., & Tamblyn, R. M. (1980). *Problem-based learning: An approach to medical education*. New York, NY: Springer Publishing.

Benner, P., Sutphen, M., Leonard, V., & Day, L. (1984/2010). *Educating nurses: A call for radical transformation*. San Francisco, CA: Jossey-Bass.

Bowen, J. L. (2006). Educational strategies to promote clinical diagnostic reasoning. *New England Journal of Medicine, 355*, 2217–2225.

Charlin, B., Mann, K., & Hansen, P. (1998). The many faces of problem-based learning: A framework for understanding and comparison. *Medical Teacher, 20*(4), 323–330.

Cornell, P., Gervis, M. T., Yates, L., & Vardaman, J. M. (2013). Improving shift report focus and consistency with the situation, background, assessment, recommendation protocol. *Journal of Nursing Administration, 43*(7/8), 422–428.

Dochy, F., Segers, M., Van den Bossche, P., & Gijbels, D. (2003). Effects of problem-based learning: A meta-analysis. *Learning and Instruction, 13*, 533–568.

Dolmans, D., Snellen-Balendong, H., Wolfhagen, I., & van der Vleuten, C. P. (1997). Seven principles of effective case design for a problem-based curriculum. *Medical Teacher, 19*(3), 185–189.

Drummond-Young, M., & Mohide, E. A. (2001). Developing problems for use in problem-based learning. In E. Rideout (Ed.), *Transforming nursing education through problem-based learning* (pp. 165–191). Sudbury, MA: Jones & Bartlett.

Durham, C. O., Fowler, T., & Kennedy, S. (2014). Teaching dual-process diagnostic reasoning to doctor of nursing practice students: Problem-based learning and the illness script. *Journal of Nursing Education, 53*(11), 646–650.

Gijbels, D., Dochy, F., Van den Bossche, P., & Segers, M. (2005). Effects of problem-based learning: A meta-analysis from the angle of assessment. *Review of Educational Research, 75*(1), 27–61.

Grabinger, R. S., & Dunlap, J. C. (1995). Rich environments for active learning: A definition. *Research in Learning Technology, 3*(2), 5–34.

Harden R. M., & Davis, M. H. (1998). The continuum of problem-based learning. *Medical Teacher, 20*(4), 317–322.

Hung, W. (2006). The 3C3R model: A conceptual framework for designing problems in PBL. *Interdisciplinary Journal of Problem-Based Learning, 1*(1), 55–77.

Hung, W. (2009). The 9-step problem design process for problem-based learning: Application of the 3C3R model. *Educational Research Review, 4*, 118–141.

Hung, W. (2011). Theory to reality: A few issues in implementing problem-based learning. *Educational Technology Research and Development, 59*, 529–552.

Larimore, W. L., & Jordan, E. V. (1995). SOAP to SNOCAMP: Improving the medical record format. *Journal of Family Practice, 41*(4), 393–398.

McCracken, R. (2015). Foreword. In N. Courtney, C. Poulsen, & C. Stylios (Eds.), *Case based teaching and learning for the 21st century* (p. viii). Faringdon, Oxfordshire, England: Libri Publishing.

Merriam, S. B. (2001). Andragogy and self-directed learning: Pillars of adult learning theory. *New Directions for Adult and Continuing Education, 89*, 3–13.

Miller, M. D. (2014). *Minds online: Teaching effectively with technology.* Cambridge, MA: Harvard University Press.

Nathanson, S. (1998). Designing problems to teach legal problem solving. *California Western Law Review, 34*(2), 325–349. Retrieved from http://scholarlycommons.law.cwsl.edu/cgi/viewcontent.cgi?article=1263&context=cwlr

Roediger, H. L., & Karpicke, J. D. (2006). The power of testing memory: Basic research and implications for educational practice. *Perspectives on Psychological Science, 1*(3), 181–210.

Rovai, A. P. (2004). A constructivist approach to online college learning. *Internet and Higher Education, 7,* 79–93.

Savin-Baden, M. (2007). *A practical guide to problem-based learning online.* New York, NY: Routledge.

Schön, D. (1983). *The reflective practitioner.* San Francisco, CA: Jossey-Bass.

Shin, I., & Kim, J. (2013). The effect of problem-based learning in nursing education: A meta-analysis. *Advances in Health Science Education, 18,* 1103–1120.

Vernon, D. T. A., & Blake, R. L. (1993, July). Does problem-based learning work? A meta-analysis of evaluative research. *Academic Medicine, 68*(7), 550–563.

Weed, L. L. (1968). Medical records that guide and teach. *New England Journal of Medicine, 278*(12), 652–657.

Wiggins, G., & McTighe, J. (2005). *Understanding by design* (2nd ed.). Alexandria, VA: Association for Supervision and Curriculum Development.

7

Writing Engaging Discussion Questions

Discussion boards are the equivalent of classroom discussions (Dereshiwsky, 2015), but afford additional opportunities for both formative and summative assessments as well as direct teaching. Possibly their best advantage over classroom discussion is that discussion boards *eliminate* the psychosocial aspects that favor articulate students who can think fast on their feet and disfavor those who are more reflective. Another drawback of classroom discussions is that not all students can voice their opinions for various reasons—they are shy or unprepared or prefer to reflect before stating their views. Or they disagree with what has been presented, yet are reticent to speak up. Some simply have nothing to add. Thus, classroom discussions often reflect somewhat of a *groupthink*.

In the online environment, a certain anonymity prevails. The visual and aural cues of smiles, eye rolling, chuckling, or sighing in response to a comment or opinion expressed are absent. Brookfield and Preskill (2005) note that students more readily share their own carefully thought-out perspective in online discussions even if they reflect an opposing view, which often makes for an interesting and engaging discussion. In addition, online discussions allow students the time to reflect upon the question, which is beneficial as participation is required and points are at stake. This opportunity to reflect fosters less pressure to conform to the groupthink, resulting in individual intellectual development and a wider range of perspectives to be considered for coconstruction of knowledge.

In this chapter, we discuss the value of online small group discussions and how to develop engaging discussion questions (DQs). This chapter walks you through the process of designing engaging DQs from an outcome-based approach. Examples of DQs are provided to give you an idea of what is possible.

ANATOMY OF A DQ

Given the variety of content in online RN to bachelor of science in nursing (BSN) and graduate nursing courses, writing a step-by-step process for faculty to follow when creating DQs that is specific enough to be useful seems to be without precedent. However, several concepts, models, theories, and sound suggestions from scholars can guide us, notably the recommendations from Benner, Sutphen, Leonard, and Day (1984/2010) to situate what we want students to learn within a context similar to how they will encounter that content in the role they aspire to. In addition, research on and decades of experience with problem-based learning (PBL) and identified characteristics of engaging DQs are also useful.

Content: Characteristics of Authentic Problems

The work of Barrows and Kelson (1996) on creating authentic cases for PBL can inform the creation of engaging DQs as well.

1. *Format*: Ill structured and messy
2. *Initial information*: Inadequate information is provided initially to solve the problem. Additional discourse and research are needed.
3. *Educational resources*: Students must engage in independent research and evaluate the reliability and value of resources they use.

To their list, I would add the following characteristics of *authentic problems*. DQs should:

- *Evoke emotions*: Recent research on memory and emotion indicates that we remember what we care about (Nairne, 2010, as cited in Miller, 2014). Starting a discussion with a video of the patient or situation involved in the problem or issue can serve to involve the area of the brain, the amygdala, where emotions arise. The more real the topic, the more involved students will become, and the more they will learn.
- *Be challenging*: DQs should be written at such a level that students will not become frustrated in composing an answer. They should be written slightly above the student's capability, but within their zone of proximal development (see Chapter 2). The challenge occurs naturally when they cannot paraphrase directly from the readings, but instead must analyze, synthesize, or evaluate what they have read in order to apply the information to the issue at hand.
- *Promote and require active learning:* Increasing student engagement is, in my experience, related to how relevant students feel the exercise is

to their future role. Perceived relevance results in students taking a more active role in their learning.

- *Promote higher order cognitive processing:* Having high expectations of students is important, as they will rise to meet these expectations. Students who will be taking online courses are already nurses who have a professional goal. I do believe they want to be challenged, but in a supportive environment where feedback helps them learn.

- *Not have one correct answer:* Some answers will be better than others, but students should *not* be able to open their text and find the answer. Fact-based questions increase cognitive load as students struggle to find something new that a classmate has not already said. This is not conducive to learning.

- *Be clearly worded:* If students cannot understand what is being asked or if the intent of the question is unclear, students will struggle with their response, become frustrated, and lose engagement with the problem.

Ross (1997) offers recommendations for *problem selection* based on experience using problems to teach. From his perspective, the problem can be selected:

- To ensure that students cover a predefined area of knowledge
- To help students learn a set of important concepts, ideas, techniques
- For its suitability for leading students to (parts of) the "field"
- For its intrinsic interest or importance
- Because it represents a typical problem faced by the profession (pp. 30–31)

Note that in the first bullet point the pesky word *cover* surfaces again. I would prefer to replace the word *cover* with *uncover*, which, according to Wiggins and McTighe (2005), "suggests finding something important in what had become hidden" (p. 230). That is truly what we want students to do. We want them to recall what they already know, think of themselves as detectives, and search out the relevant information needed to answer the questions posed. These recommendations align with the call for transformation of nursing education that you will recall include learning within context, integration of knowing and doing, and using the thought processes necessary for the role.

When talking about online discussions, Brookfield and Preskill wrote (2005):

Discussion is not particularly effective for disclosing new facts or for arguing over something that can be checked out by consulting an almanac or dictionary. Discussion *is* ideal, however, for exploring complex ideas and entertaining multiple perspectives. It is almost never suitable for reaching definitive solutions or putting forward a single, indisputable answer. (p. 236)

When writing DQs, as faculty we know what it is we want students to learn from a question. We could tell them in a lecture what they *need to learn*. However, research (Bransford, Brown, & Cocking, 1999) has shown that lecturing supports surface learning (Chapter 1) that is quickly forgotten because information is presented without context. Our goal is to present an authentic problem or issue embedded within a context that students will recognize in order to uncover the essence of what is to be learned. We want to support development of "habits of thought" that will serve them throughout their careers.

Content Considerations

A word of caution is in order when beginning to consider content for your course. The process of DQ development for nonclinical courses requires a specific focus due to the breadth of content available that can seemingly push faculty toward teaching habits that are undesirable from a constructivist, learner-centered perspective. What I am referring to is the idea faculty sometimes have that they must teach everything there is to know about a topic in *one* course. This is counterproductive.

Recall from the work of Wiggins and McTighe (2005) that coverage is not the best approach, and is in fact considered one of the "twin sins" of instructional design. As faculty, we must face reality and understand that if our students are to learn *anything*, not *everything* about the topic can be taught (Locher, 2004). Bransford et al. (1999) explained this phenomenon: "curricula that emphasize breadth of knowledge may prevent effective organization of knowledge because there is not enough time to learn anything in depth" (p. 49). Sacrificing breadth of content so that students learn the essential content in a deep, as opposed to surface, manner (see Chapter 1) and learn for *understanding* (see Chapter 3) is the best approach. So, the key is to determine what content is *essential* for students to learn (*must know*) because it will be put to use in their future role. Separate that from content that is simply *nice to know* and content that, if taught, will quickly be forgotten as students will most likely not use it. So, the question is, What knowledge is essential for students to function effectively in their future role that must be learned from *this* course? Remember your new mantra: *outcomes*.

Thoughts on Context

From Benner and colleagues (1984/2010) comes the challenge to transform nursing education, which includes learning within an authentic context, integration of clinical and classroom teaching, and formation within the role that should be at the foundation of our approach to question development and teaching in general. DQs should be grounded in a context that reflects the professional role and affords practice in thinking like a professional nurse, nurse practitioner (NP), researcher, administrator, or educator. Tanner (2009) refers to this practice as developing *habits of thought,* which means "critically evaluating the evidence supporting alternative choices, reflecting on one's reasoning processes and self-correcting, understanding patient's experiences, identifying salient aspects of a situation, making clinical judgments in specific situations, and modifying one's approach in light of the patient's responses" (p. 299). Although this quote is obviously written from a clinical context, the type of thinking or habits of thought can be applied to nonclinical nursing roles as well.

From my experience, students, even with nursing experience, too readily take new information and data at face value without question or an attempt to seek validation. These habits of thought Tanner refers to are best developed through guided problem-solving practice in a safe environment where students not only have feedback, coaching, and support from faculty, but also the opportunity to observe experienced faculty (and more experienced classmates) model the expert's thought processes, which is akin to the experience of cognitive apprenticeship (Collins, Brown, & Newman, 1984); also see Chapter 2).

The Role of Context

Must all DQs include context? What is wrong with simply asking a question? Questions asked out of context may leave the student wondering, *Why should I care about this? So what?* Remember the tenets of andragogy that adults are independent learners who have accumulated rich life experiences who prefer to apply what they are learning to their changing social role (i.e., a new career) (Merriam, 2001). In addition, context helps add additional cues for retrieval. Brown, Roediger, and McDaniel (2014) made the point that:

> How readily you can recall knowledge from your internal archives is determined by context, by recent use, and by the number and vividness of cues that you have linked to the knowledge and can call on to help bring it forth. (p. 76)

Because there is a mismatch between the vast amounts of data our brains can store compared to the finite ability to cue the memories, it makes sense to help provide a context whenever possible to help students retrieve the content when it is needed in their new roles. Keep in mind that most, if not all, questions aimed to satisfy learning outcomes could be presented within context, even questions on statistics, statistical methods, and concepts related to research. What is required is a bit of imagination and creativity. Asking yourself, *Why does the student need to know this?*, may help uncover an appropriate context.

FOCUSING ON OUTCOMES

From the Backward Design process, I hope your new mantra is *outcomes* and that the question you ask yourselves when planning instruction is: *What are the desired learning outcomes?* This is the place to begin when writing DQs. A look at the objectives for the course is the best place to start, paying particular attention to the domain and level of verb used. If the objectives are broadly written, they may not provide enough information to drill down to the actual DQs. A task analysis of the objective as discussed in Chapter 8 may help you understand the particular knowledge, skills, and attitudes that students must learn in your course. The steps of a task analysis used to determine the knowledge and skills necessary to meet an objective are listed in Box 7.1.

Perhaps an example will help. In the Online Methodologies course I taught, one of the content areas was facilitating online discussions. Students read about the theory and strategies of facilitation, but my goal was for each of them to actually facilitate a discussion. The objective for the course related to this content was: At the end of the course, students will be able to successfully *demonstrate* effective facilitation strategies. This objective is

---

BOX 7.1
STEPS OF A TASK ANALYSIS OF AN OBJECTIVE

1. Determine the domain of the objective (cognitive, psychomotor, or affective).
2. Determine the level of performance desired (measurable verb in the objective).
3. Make a list of knowledge, skills, and attitudes (abilities) necessary to meet the objective. Questions to help with this step are:
   a. How will this content reveal itself to solve problems?
   b. What are common problems students might later encounter that are related to this content?
   c. What is the context in which these problems might occur?
   d. What prerequisite knowledge, skills, and attitudes should be brought to mind to help them build mental models?
4. Identify an authentic problem and situation (context) that would require the application of the identified abilities.

written in the cognitive domain, application level. One of my perspectives on teaching is that I want to combine *knowing* and *doing* whenever possible in order to make the content become real for the student.

To assess this objective, I planned to have each student facilitate one discussion in the course. I set up a discussion board for the leaders of each discussion—one from each group—to work on and to ultimately write the DQ that all groups would tackle for their assigned module. I lurked in the background of these decision-making discussions and provided guidance when necessary. What I wanted students to experience when they facilitated a discussion was keeping the discussion going, using various facilitative techniques to support learning, such as providing encouragement, requesting clarification, Socratic questioning, metacognitive questioning, and so on (all included in Chapter 11). Thus, the actual question they created was about the topic for the module. For this example, I will use the topic of teaching with cases.

The objective: At the end of the course, students will be able to successfully demonstrate effective facilitation strategies.

- Domain: Cognitive
- Level of performance: Application
- Knowledge, skills, and attitudes
  - Content knowledge of the topic at hand, teaching with cases, and knowledge of facilitation strategies.
  - The skill of successfully using these strategies (being able to apply them) by choosing the right words to promote participation and move the discussion forward.
  - To portray a supportive attitude for their "learners."
  - To recognize what is occurring in the discussion and in each student's posts such as nonsubstantive posts, superficial response to classmates that reiterates rather than continues the discourse, or a series of monologues and not really a discussion and deal with them.
- Authentic problem: Having students lead a discussion of their peers on the authentic of teaching with cases.

I hope you can see where taking the time to go through this process will help you gain clarity on desired outcomes that will assess the objective and offer some idea of what the DQ will be about.

WRITING DQs

DQs are written in somewhat of a story format that includes an authentic *context* that mimics the situation in which students will encounter the *content* in their future role. The content is introduced in the form of an issue, dilemma, or problem to be solved that includes relevant information and possibly extraneous information to make the question *messy* and realistic. I have used the term *foreground content* when referring to the main content area and the additional relevant or irrelevant content is referred to as *background information*, which helps to create the context of the DQ. I have found that differentiating content using these naming conventions is helpful, especially if a team is writing the DQs. This content was covered in Chapter 6 under section Core Components: The Three Cs, but will be revisited here and customized to writing DQs.

Foreground Content

I consider the problem to be solved and other relevant information as the foreground portion of the DQ. Foreground content includes information that frames the problem or dilemma and is the starting point for inquiry.

Background Information

Background information is the scene that helps to create a real-life scenario around the foreground content. Like developing a scene for a movie, the background information creates context. It is also what will make a DQ *ill structured* or *messy*. The background may include relevant, irrelevant, and frankly unnecessary information to solve the problem or issue, but it presents the content in such a way that the student can *see* and *feel* that it is relevant and real. The background content may not be essential to solving the problem at hand, but may include subproblems students should identify and plan for, as they may impact the path taken toward solution or resolution.

The foreground content should pose a problem that the background information complicates and/or defines, such as barriers, limitations, and constraints that must be understood and considered. The question, either implied or directly asked, must stretch the student's current ability, challenge, and engage him or her, but the solution or resolution must be achievable with effort. What we want to do is create a *desirable difficulty*.

Professional Context

Separate from the background information is the professional context in which the problem will occur. To some degree, the program in which the student is enrolled dictates the professional context. For example, NP students with family, adult/geriatrics, some pediatrics, or women's health foci will typically find jobs in primary care settings such as clinics or physicians' offices. The acute care NP, on the other hand, will most likely work in a hospital. Therefore, the professional context for the cases they will discuss should reflect the particular role they are studying for. This is a slightly different consideration than what you would include in the background information. For example, in a policy course as part of a doctor of nursing practice (DNP) program, you may want students to get involved with current pending legislation in their respective cities. Even though they are family nurse practitioner (FNP) students, for example, the professional context may be at the local nurses' association headquarters where they are collaborating to develop a plan to block a specific bill. This type of context adds realism to the case and will help to engage students.

THE ROLE OF EFFORT IN LEARNING

Desirable Difficulties

The educational goal when creating DQs is to incorporate *desirable difficulties,* to borrow a term from cognitive psychology. Desirable difficulties were described by Bjork and Bjork (2011) as conditions of instruction that are designed to *slow the rate of learning* that lead to long-term retention and transfer. I realize that seems completely counterintuitive, but research has shown that rapid learning through repetition and rereading, in other words, to learn for the short term to pass a test or what is termed *massed study* (cramming), is less effective than effortful learning by varying the conditions of practice (Bjork & Bjork, 2011; Kerfoot, 2009; Kerfoot et al., 2010; Roediger & Karpicke, 2006). *Effort* is created through spaced study, interleaving, and retrieval practice, all discussed in Chapter 1. According to Bjork and Bjork (2011):

> Desirable difficulties, versus the array of undesirable difficulties, are desirable because they trigger encoding and retrieval processes that support learning, comprehension, and remembering. If, however, the learner does not have the background knowledge or skills to respond to them successfully, they become undesirable difficulties. (p. 58)

So, to some degree wrestling with a DQ to synthesize, analyze, and evaluate information and successfully apply it to the issue at hand is a function of the students' prior knowledge and their ability to persist. Thus, you want to challenge students with the DQ, a problem in a context that will be recognized as authentic by the student, in such a way that the student can draw on prior knowledge. In small group online discussions, students will post their thoughts based on synthesis of the readings, read the posts of others, and refine their position through discourse and coconstruction of knowledge.

Knowledge Generation

The studies on the testing effect initially used recall questions, such as fill in the blank, and found them to improve learning and transfer (Roediger & Karpicke, 2006). This type of question requires that students *generate* answers, which necessitates retrieval from long-term memory and is more beneficial to learning than being told the answer or looking it up (Bjork & Bjork, 2011). The researchers felt that retrieval strengthened the cues that were linked to the memory and incorporating a context helped to create additional cues. The interesting and counterintuitive part of this is the role of forgetting. According to Brown, Roediger, and McDaniel (2014), "the more effort required to retrieve (or, in effect, relearn) something, the better you learn it. In other words, the more you've forgotten about a topic, the more effective relearning will be in shaping your permanent knowledge" (p. 81).

I think this may be why online discussions are a promising way to learn, as they include all the components to improve long-term memory and transfer supported by cognitive science research. Students are required to generate their responses and revisit them after a lapse of time after classmates and faculty have responded to their posts (spaced study). This requires retrieval of information as they have most likely been studying other content in the meantime for another course. This describes interleaving (Chapter 1). In effect, discussions over a 2-week time frame are a version of spaced study combined with the retrieval effect and interleaving that have the potential to support long-term learning and transfer.

Must All Online Courses Include DQs?

This is a good question to consider when planning assessments and teaching methods for an online course. Some courses are built around the various phases of completing the capstone writing project, particularly the dissertation in the PhD program and the evidence-based improvement project in the DNP program. In this type of situation, sections of the final paper are due at intervals throughout the course so that faculty can provide in-depth, individual feedback to students. This is a time-intensive process that is very beneficial for students in terms of individual learning. When this is the focus of a course, discussions may be busywork for students (and you).

If critiquing others' work is an objective for the course, pairing students in a discussion forum to provide feedback on each other's work may be a good pedagogical decision. However, students should be matched strategically based on the topic of their dissertations or projects, if possible. I would avoid setting up discussion boards with five or so students in each and having them critique others work. This approach can be cumbersome for faculty to monitor, adding busywork, and increasing cognitive load for students, as they must take time to understand what they are reading, which may require additional research before they can critique it. If a wiki option is available in the learning management system (LMS), students can write comments within their classmate's paper in a different-colored font and can edit their own work as they go. In addition, you can provide feedback and eventually grade the work within the wiki as well, saving the step of downloading a paper that is separated from the peer assessment. More about the benefit of using a wiki appears in Chapter 12.

DECONSTRUCTING EXPERT KNOWLEDGE

I think the reason that articulating how to write DQs is so difficult relates to the essence of how knowledge is stored in cognitive structures by experts (Benner, 1984/2001). After all, intuition is difficult to deconstruct. Experts, when compared to novices, have a larger repertoire of *domain* (content) knowledge, which is stored more effectively and efficiently as complex mental models and can be more readily retrieved. Experts also have acquired experience or skill in using that domain knowledge and often do so intuitively. However, as experts, this knowledge is stored in *condition* (stimulus)–*action* (response) modules (Larkin, 1979, as cited in Stepich, 1991) that may be difficult to disentangle. So, basically writing DQs requires the expert to break down sophisticated cognitive knowledge structures into the component parts—domain knowledge (*knowing that*) and procedural knowledge (*knowing how*)—in order to map the problem and process inherent in a DQ.

Those who teach in nursing are also required to practice, conduct research, and/or write grants in addition to their many other faculty responsibilities. Thus, creative time is limited for readying the next semester's course and developing rich and engaging DQs. By providing various authors' and educators' unique thoughts on writing DQs, it is my hope that one or more will resonate with you to assist in the process of discussion board question development.

MAPPING DISCUSSIONS

DQ Development Worksheet

The process of identifying essential content may be intuitive for faculty who are content experts in the field. However, for many it is a struggle. DQs can be written as standalone questions or build on each other to create a final assignment, such as an individual or group project.

I have provided four examples of DQ development in various types of nursing courses. This DQ development worksheet, shown in Exhibits 7.1 through 7.4, allows you to associate the issue for discussion with the objective(s) being assessed, foreground content, background information (context), and the professional context. I would recommend copying and pasting the objectives for the course at the top so you can refer to them as you write. Because all objectives must be assessed, this format will help you create DQs to assess specific objectives and track your progress.

Exhibits 7.1 through 7.4 are examples of using the DQ development worksheet to construct DQ from the course objectives for various levels and types of nursing courses. An example of a DQ is included with each worksheet.

I have developed a Discussion Question Development Worksheet as a Word document that you can use as a template to align the elements when writing a DQ. Template 7.1 can be found in the Appendix as well as on the Springer website for download.

- Exhibit 7.1: an example from a PhD-level course, Ethics in Research
- Exhibit 7.2: an example from an RN–BSN course, Population Health
- Exhibit 7.3: an example from a PhD- or DNP-level, nonclinical course, Health Care Policy
- Exhibit 7.4: an example from an NP course, Patient Care Management

The DQ Map for the Course

The final step I have found useful is to create a smaller document from the DQ development worksheet that I call the DQ map for the course. Included in this document are the DQs by module, the content I expect students to discuss, and the connections I want them to make. This serves as a handy resource when facilitating discussions to help keep me focused on the intent and the desired learning outcomes of each DQ. An example of the DQ map for the DQ shown in Exhibit 7.4, the clinical NP case DQ, is shown in Exhibit 7.5. A template for the DQ map (Template 7.5) can be found in the Appendix. The customizable template can also be downloaded from the Springer website.

EXHIBIT 7.1

PhD Discussion Question Development Worksheet

Name of course: Ethics in Research
Program of study: PhD
Numbered objectives for course:

1. Differentiate ethical and unethical aspects of conducting research.
2. Defend options to protect vulnerable populations when planning for and conducting research.
3. Assess methods to recruit research subjects with consideration to vulnerability, equity, inclusion, and avoidance of bias.
4. Correlate aspects of vulnerability with ethical decisions in research.

DQ	Problem or Issue	Foreground Content	Background Content	Professional Context	Objective Number Assessed
1	Recognize the variety of potentially unethical requests regarding various aspects of research, including subjects. Issue: remaining objective and impartial when making decisions based on ethics	Researchers, some of whom are known to the facility and others who are new, present ideas for research. Some aspects of the ideas presented are ethical, some not.	Funding is down for the facility and is desperately needed to continue operations. A few employees will need to be let go unless more research dollars are soon obtained.	Committee to vet potential research in a college of nursing, hospital, or outpatient facility. A different context could be used for each discussion group.	1, 2, 3
2	Knowledge base from which to defend decisions	Same as DQ 1	Same as DQ 1	Same as DQ 1	2

(continued)

EXHIBIT 7.1

PhD Discussion Question Development Worksheet (*continued*)

DQ	Problem or Issue	Foreground Content	Background Content	Professional Context	Objective Number Assessed
3	Knowledge base related to vulnerability, equity, inclusion, and avoidance of bias in order to determine ethical vs. unethical means of recruiting subjects	Same as DQ 1, except the committee will be evaluating a written research proposal.	Committee members have strong personalities and often disagree. Some are more concerned with "doing the right thing" and others find the committee meetings laborious and want decisions made quickly.	Members of institutional review board in hospital, HMO, or VA psychiatric clinic or other outpatient facility; a different context could be used for each discussion group	3
4	Definition of vulnerable populations and terms used in the Belmont Report	The PI of a research study is anxious to enroll patients in his study. He puts pressure on the clinical research coordinator and research assistant to do so.	The PI, clinical research coordinator, and research assistant are not in agreement about how to recruit patients for the study even though protocols are in place.	A privately owned psychiatric facility	1–4

DQ, discussion question; HMO, health maintenance organization; PI, principal investigator; VA, Veterans Affairs.
Discussion question for Objective No. 4.

Dr. Smith is the PI of a research study to test the use of cannabis in treating psychotic symptoms in patients with schizophrenia. He is anxious to start the project as the deadline looms for the first required progress report. He is putting pressure on Mary Smith, RN, the clinical research coordinator who is also his wife, and Jane Jones, the research assistant whose responsibility is to enroll patients in the study. They have decided to recruit subjects from the local, private psychiatric facility owned by Dr. Smith where 25 patients with paranoid schizophrenia who would otherwise be homeless are housed and treated based on Kendra's law. Dr. Smith has indicated to Mary and Jane that he expects them to sign up all 25 patients for this study the next day. Although Jane enthusiastically agrees to do so, Mary has reservations. What would you do if you were Mary? Include rationales for your decision based on ethical considerations.

Note: See the Appendix for a blank version of this template.

EXHIBIT 7.2
RN to Bachelor of Science in Nursing (BSN) Discussion Question
Development Worksheet

Name of course: Population Health
Program of study: RN–BSN
Numbered objectives for course:

1. Assess a community using an epidemiological approach for a need
   related to health promotion, disease prevention, or environmental
   health that can be impacted by a nursing intervention.
2. Analyze epidemiological and other data from a community assessment
   to guide development of nursing interventions.
3. Determine the appropriate evidence-based nursing interventions based
   on epidemiological principles for level of need; individual, community,
   or population.
4. Demonstrate professional communication skills when presenting
   assessment findings, supportive documentation, the program plan, and
   evaluation strategies to community partners.

Problem or issue: Most likely students are accustomed to working within an
acute care setting. Consequently, much of this content and approach to popu-
lation-focused care will be new.

Foreground content: Provide students with a list of the components of a community assessment that you want them to address.

Background content: Epidemiological and community health care concepts
and principles

Professional context: Mega context (for entire course)—Because this course is
online and students may reside in a variety of geographic areas, a virtual community will need to be used, perhaps one for each discussion group in the course.
The other option would be to choose one community, but have the groups
obtain approval from you as to which need they plan to address, so that each
group will address a different need. Faculty should choose a rural community or
communities that have accessible data from the local health departments for
students to work with. Other necessary data about the community should be
available on the web. The community assessment can be done using Google
Maps or other online mapping software that provides an overview of the com-
munity- and street-level views.

Subcontext—Grant money has become available for community-level demonstration projects for health promotion, disease prevention, or environmental
health–related projects. The students are part of the committee to determine
the greatest need in the community. The task for this committee is to identify
the most important need and provide rationales for the decision, justify the

(continued)

EXHIBIT 7.2
RN to Bachelor of Science in Nursing (BSN) Discussion Question
Development Worksheet (*continued*)

need with available community data, identify potential stakeholders and their roles, develop a workable plan to address the need, and create a professional presentation for a community meeting.

Discussions: This type of activity will not require discussions and will address all course objectives. Because a group project presentation is the deliverable that will come out of this small group project, biweekly discussions are not necessary. Instead, create online discussion areas where each group of students can discuss what they are doing in the various steps of the community population health project so that you can monitor their progress and provide feedback, direction, and/or correction. Assign due dates for various phases of the project to keep them on track and provide feedback along the way. If a wiki is available within the learning management system (Moodle, Blackboard, etc.), students can organize the presentation there. GoogleDrive is another option using Word or PowerPoint software. Either way, you can monitor their activity and watch the level of participation of all students. Initially, ask them to each use a different-colored font to monitor individual participation. They can change the font when the presentation is completed, and you have assessed participation.

Note: See the Appendix for a blank version of this template.

EXHIBIT 7.3

Nonclinical Course Discussion Question Development Worksheet

Name of course: Health Care Policy
Program of study: DNP or PhD

Numbered objectives for course:

1. Determine characteristics of effective nursing leaders and advocates.
2. Analyze health policies from a variety of perspectives, including that of consumers, health care professionals, health care organizations, and other potential stakeholders.
3. Apply health services theory and best evidence to create a new policy or revise an existing one.
4. Devise a plan for a new health care policy or revision of an existing policy utilizing knowledge of health policy and/or health services theory, best practices, health care financing, and ethical comportment.
5. Demonstrate effective leadership characteristics and strategies when presenting the new or revised health care policy to stakeholders.

DQ	Problem or Issue	Foreground Content	Background Content	Professional Context	Objective Number Assessed
1	A health care policy needs to be changed or revised. An interprofessional committee has been appointed by the administration, placing a nurse in charge.	Nurse takes the leadership role over an interprofessional committee to assess, create, and sell the policy change to stakeholders. Policy is chosen.	In addition to the chair, who is a nurse, the members of the interprofessional group include two physicians, a physical therapist, occupational therapist, social worker, and nursing administrator.	Mega context for course—Several settings can be used: hospital, outpatient clinic, and/or nursing organization. You may want to use a different context for each discussion group.	1, 5

(continued)

EXHIBIT 7.3

Nonclinical Course Discussion Question Development Worksheet (*continued*)

DQ	Problem or Issue	Foreground Content	Background Content	Professional Context	Objective Number Assessed
2	Analyzing a policy from various perspectives.	The leader assigns tasks to the group to analyze the policy from various perspectives. Students should be assigned roles of the various professionals in the group.	Same as DQ 1	Same as DQ 1	2, 5
3	The group discusses available evidence and how it applies to changing the policy.	Evidence is applied to the policy to convince stakeholders.	Same as DQ 1	Same as DQ 1	3, 5
4	Develop the new policy.	Policy is developed.	Same as DQ 1	Same as DQ 1	4, 5
5	Presentation appropriate to the level of stakeholders needs to be developed.	Leader assigned to orchestrate the presentation.	Same as DQ 1	Same as DQ 1	5

DNP, doctor of nursing practice; DQ, discussion question.

You have been assigned to lead an interprofessional committee to revise a current health care policy. Options for discussion within the small groups are:

1. The NPs in your state cannot function autonomously. They are required to have a "supervising" physician who will review a subset of medical records each month and sign-off on protocols they work under. This committee is assigned to present a revision to this policy to the legislature.

2. In the assisted living facility, patients 65 years of age and older with chronic indwelling urinary catheters have an unusually high incidence of urinary tract infections using the current procedures of catheter care. The committee has been assigned to look into why this is occurring and make recommendations for changes in the policy.

3. You are a health care consultant who has been hired by a Fortune 500 company to lead a committee to research the need and support for and financial benefit of changing employee health care coverage to *exclude* contraceptive services, including medications, devices, and surgery. The demographics of the employees in this company show that 75% of the employees are younger than 40 years of age, with 60% of that group being female.

4. You have been asked to chair an interprofessional committee to improve the transition for patients from hospital to home, especially access to uninterrupted health care, sharing of information among and between various health care providers, access to medications and needed devices, and to assess changes in readmission rates. Current data suggest a high readmission rate, and the reasons seem to be related to the issues mentioned previously. No policy exists currently, so one will need to be created.

In order for you to assess Objective 5, you will need to observe the conversation, so I recommend setting up discussion boards or using a wiki. Collaborative writing is best done in a wiki or GoogleDrive so you can monitor contributions from each student, which is easily done if each student in the small group uses a different-colored font.

The new policy must be presented to the stakeholders. This can be a group deliverable using GoogleDrive or a wiki. If a verbal presentation is desired, students can create a podcast to accompany PowerPoint slides or do a voice-over PowerPoint that can be converted to a YouTube video.

Note: See the Appendix for a blank version of this template.

EXHIBIT 7.4

NP Discussion Question Development Worksheet

Name of course: Patient Care Management
Program of study: DNP
Numbered objectives for course:

1. Combine knowledge of pathophysiology, pharmacotherapeutics, nursing science, and best evidence, including emerging genetic and genomic evidence to assess, evaluate, diagnose, and manage patients with episodic, chronic, and comorbid behavioral illnesses in the outpatient setting.
2. Assess unique patient variables, such as age, gender, and family history, to develop a patient-centric plan for health promotion and disease prevention.
3. Apply the Code of Ethics for Nurses to all aspects of professional nursing practice.

DQ	Problem or Issue	Foreground Content	Background Content	Professional Context	Objective Number Assessed
1	A sign or symptom that can be caused by the same body system or multiple systems	Brief chief complaint that includes the gender and age of the patient and any additional information necessary for students to arrive at potential causal hypotheses.	Add comorbidities, social issues, implications from the family history, ethical issues, and classes of medications for comorbidities.	Outpatient setting	1–3

| 2 | Acting ethically | Ethical dilemma with a patient or other professional. For example, prescribing a controlled substance for a family member. | A good sob story can be created in which this type of behavior may seem allowable. | Same as above | 3 |

DNP, doctor of nursing practice; DQ, discussion question; NP, nurse practitioner. Discussion question to assess all objectives.

Marie, an 80-year-old woman, is brought to your office by her daughter, who complains her mother has "not seemed quite right" for the past week. Marie is able to answer all your questions and seems quite cognitively intact. You also notice that the daughter seems disinterested in the conversation, and her speech seems somewhat slowed and her pupils are dilated. When Marie is helped to the bathroom by your assistant to leave a urine specimen, the daughter approaches you to ask you to declare her mother mentally incompetent so she can assume charge of her financial affairs.

Note: See the Appendix for a blank version of this template.

EXHIBIT 7.5
Discussion Question Map Example

This coincides with the DQ worksheet, Exhibit 7.4.

Module 3	
DQ: Marie, an 80-year-old woman, is brought to your office by her daughter, who complains her mother has "not seemed quite right" for the past week. Marie is able to answer all your questions and seems quite cognitively intact. You also notice that the daughter seems disinterested in the conversation, and her speech seems somewhat slowed and her pupils are dilated. When Marie is helped to the bathroom by your assistant to leave a urine specimen, the daughter approaches you to ask you to declare her mother mentally incompetent so she can assume charge of her financial affairs.	
Content	**Connections**
Working hypotheses—delirium, thyroid issue, anemia, hyponatremia, medication side effect	Short-term mental changes are delirium until proven otherwise.
History—symptoms of infection; UTI, pneumonia; signs of physical abuse or neglect	Other family members may need to be interviewed.
Exam—general appearance, HEENT, cardiac, pulmonary, neuro exam including MMSE, relationship with daughter	Daughter may have hidden agenda. Concern for mental and/or physical abuse.
Lab—urinalysis in office, lab—consider CBC, TSH, electrolytes. Consider CXR depending on findings on exam	Will need short-term plan and perhaps a plan for the patient's safety until this can be sorted out.
Plan to include	

CBC, complete blood count; CXR, chest x-ray; DQ, discussion question; HEENT, head, eyes, ears, nose, throat; MMSE, Mini-Mental State Examination; TSH, thyroid-stimulating hormone; UTI, urinary tract infection.

Note: See the Appendix for a blank version of this template.

THE TAKE-AWAY

Writing engaging DQs starts with the desired learning outcomes specified in the objectives for the course. Key to creating engaging questions is to choose problems and frame them with an authentic context to mimic those that students are most likely to encounter in their future role. It is important that students be required to generate knowledge in the process of synthesizing the literature and writing their perspective, as opposed to being able to open their textbook and find the answer. Your goal is to create a desirable difficulty for your students when they wrestle with these questions in order to slow learning and make it more effortful—characteristics of learning that cognitive science research has found to be linked to long-term retention and transfer. Mapping the questions throughout the course to the objectives before the course begins will ensure that the objectives are assessed and the questions build on one another to promote the development of complex mental models.

REFERENCES

Barrows, H., & Kelson, A. (1996). *Designing a PBL problem*. Unpublished manuscript.

Benner, P. (1984/2001). *From novice to expert: Excellence and power in clinical nursing practice*. Upper Saddle River, NJ: Prentice Hall Health. [Commemorative edition. Original work published 1984]

Benner, P., Sutphen, M., Leonard, V., & Day, L. (1984/2010). *Educating nurses: A call for radical transformation*. San Francisco, CA: Jossey-Bass.

Bjork, E. L., & Bjork, R. A. (2011). Making things hard on yourself, but in a good way: Creating desirable difficulties to enhance learning. In M. A. Gernsbacher, R. W. Pew, L. M. Hough, & J. R. Pomerantz (Eds.), *Psychology and the real world: Essays illustrating fundamental contributions to society* (pp. 56–64). New York, NY: Worth.

Bransford, J. D., Brown, A. L., & Cocking, R. R. (1999). *How people learn: Brain, mind, experience, and school*. Washington, DC: National Academies Press.

Brookfield, S. D., & Preskill, S. (2005). *Discussion as a way of teaching: Tools and techniques for democratic classrooms* (2nd ed.). San Francisco, CA: Jossey-Bass.

Brown, P. C., Roediger, H. L., III, & McDaniel, M. A. (2014). *Make it stick: The science of successful learning*. Cambridge, MA: Belknap Press.

Collins, A., Brown, J. S., & Newman, S. E. (1984). Cognitive apprenticeship: Teaching the craft of reading, writing, and mathematics. In L. B. Resnick (Ed.), *Knowing, learning, and instruction: Essays in honor of Robert Glaser* (pp. 453–494). Hillside, NJ: Lawrence Erlbaum.

Dereshiwsky, M. I. (2015). Building successful student learning experiences online. In R. Papa (Ed.), *Media rich instruction: Connecting curriculum to all learners*, (pp. 49–66). New York, NY: Springer.

Kerfoot, B. P. (2009). Learning benefits of on-line spaced education persist for 2 years. *Journal of Urology, 181*, 2671–2673.

Kerfoot, B. P., Baker, H., Pangaro, L., Agarwal, K., Taffet, G., Mechaber, A. J., & Armstrong, E. G. (2012). An online spaced-education game to teach and assess medical students: A multi-institutional prospective trial. *Academic Medicine, 87*(10), 1443–1449.

Merriam, S. B. (2001). Andragogy and self-directed learning: Pillars of adult learning theory. *New Directions for Adult and Continuing Education, 89*, 3–13.

Miller, M. D. (2014). *Minds online: Teaching effectively with technology*. Cambridge, MA: Harvard University Press.

Locher, D. (2004). When teaching less is more. *Teaching Professor, 18*(9), 2–6.

Roediger, H. L., & Karpicke, J. D. (2006). The power of testing memory: Basic research and implications for educational practice. *Perspectives on Psychological Science, 1*(3), 181–210.

Ross, B. (1997). Towards a framework for problem-based curricula. In D. Boud & G. Feletti (Eds.), *The Challenge of Problem-based Learning* (pp. 28–35). New York, NY: Kogan Page. Retrieved from https://books.google.com/books?id=zvyBq6 k6tWUC&q=ross#v=snippet&q=ross&f=false

Stepich, D. (1991). From novice to expert: Implications for instructional design. *Performance & Instruction, 30*(6), 13–17.

Tanner, C. A. (2009). The case for cases: A pedagogy for developing habits of thought [Editorial]. *Journal of Nursing Education, 48*(6), 299–300.

Wiggins, G., & McTighe, J. (2005). *Understanding by design* (2nd ed.). Alexandria, VA: Association for Supervision and Curriculum Development.

8

Effective Online Testing With Multiple-Choice Questions

Tests and quizzes have been the mainstay of summative assessment in nursing education for decades. Using quizzes for *formative* assessment is, perhaps, more in line with a constructivist paradigm and exploits the testing effect. This chapter is about testing with multiple-choice questions (MCQs), how to write MCQs at various levels of Bloom's taxonomy, and the value of frequent formative assessment from a cognitive science perspective. Although assessing higher cognitive functions and abilities is key to promoting deep learning and transforming nursing education, assessing facts and understandings is of value as well to identify students' zone of proximal development (ZPD).

The goal of higher education is transfer of knowledge from the classroom to new domains that include dealing with life's challenges and functioning effectively in the workplace (Carpenter, 2012; Mayer, 1998; Merriam & Leahy, 2005). This requires that students attend to the lesson, remember what they have learned, and are able to recall the information when needed. Our goal as educators should be to teach with long-term retention and transfer in mind, and the type of teaching and assessment strategies that best accomplish this may surprise you.

MCQs—FORM AND FORMAT

Anatomy of a Test Item

An MCQ contains a *stem* and *options*, which include the correct answer and two or more distractors. The stem, which can range in length from a few words to a case containing relevant and extraneous information, comprises the question or what requires an answer (Haladyna, 2004).

Writing distractors is challenging and undoubtedly the most difficult part of creating an MCQ. Haladyna (2004) recommends that distractors should *not* stand out as different from the correct answer in terms of length, grammatical form, style, or tone. They must all be plausible in that they represent errors in learning or common mistakes made. Distractors should not be arbitrary or humorous, and they must be *clearly* incorrect answers. From a psychometric perspective, distractors are discussed in terms of functioning and nonfunctioning. A functioning distractor is one that is plausible and chosen by more than 5% of the examinees (Wakefield, 1958, as cited in Rodriguez, 2005). The value of having well-written distractors is that they serve to increase the difficulty of the item and discriminate among students (Kilgour & Tayyaba, 2015).

Controversy exists as to the best number of distractors for an MCQ. However, given that functioning distractors are difficult to write, the typical four-option approach, which consists of the correct answer plus three distractors, often leaves the item writer struggling to come up with a plausible third distractor. Thus, the recommendation based on decades of research is for only two distractors (Haladyna, 2004; Haladyna & Downing, 1993; Kilgour & Tayyaba, 2015; Rodriquez, 2005).

Controversy also exists as to whether every question on the test must have the same number of options. Some feel that the number can vary (Nitko & Brookhart, 2011, as cited in Oermann & Gaberson, 2014). Their perspective focuses on writing plausible distractors for each question; if only two can be written, then the item should contain three options. Conversely, if three plausible distractors can be written, the item will include four options. I have learned from experience in giving exams online that if most questions include four options and suddenly a question appears with three, students become concerned that an option has been inadvertently omitted from the test. Although this issue can be readily cleared up in a classroom, it becomes a problem online. If the test is timed, students have only one opportunity to take it, and if they have a question at 2 a.m. when they are taking the test, most likely you will not available by phone or e-mail to answer. I think the best practice is to follow the research recommendations and use three options for all questions. Alternatively, if questions in a test contain varied number of options, this can be mentioned in the instructions at the beginning of the test or at the end of the stem on that question. Although some may argue that a three-option question does not reflect certification exam format or contribute to increased reliability and validity, it does allow for a greater number of questions to be included in the test as students have less to read, thus potentially negating the concerns.

MCQ Formats

Conventional Format

MCQs can take various forms, but the most widely accepted and easiest for students to comprehend is considered the conventional format. In this format, a complete question or statement is made in the stem, ending in a period or question mark. No blank spaces exist within the question stem that students must fill in by selecting one of the options, nor does the stem require one of the options to complete the thought. The latter format, called the *completion* format, requires that students remember the stem while they read through the options. If the stem is lengthy and their memory fails, they must return to the stem, reread it, and reread the options (Haladyna, 2004). This slows down the test-taking process, which faculty must take into consideration when determining the number of questions to include on a test. Keep in mind that the more questions an exam contains, the more reliable and potentially valid the test will prove to be (Schneid, Armour, Park, Yudkowsky, & Bordage, 2014). Although learning management system (LMS) software will allow various question formats, writing MCQs in the conventional format will create a more efficient test.

Context-Dependent Sets

Another type of MCQ that often appears on certification exams is the context-dependent set, which consists of a case and several questions that relate to the case. This type of question has the ability to measure higher cognitive reasoning, which is so important in nursing education (Oermann & Gaberson, 2014).

Cases for context-dependent sets should include a setting (the context) that is relevant to the students' future role. Multiple questions can be based on the case and can run the gambit of the domains and levels of the three taxonomies depending upon what is to be assessed. The more *irrelevant* information included in the case, the greater the cognitive activity required to identify salient data and the more time students will need to read them.

Although the context-dependent item is rather easy to accommodate on a paper-and-pencil test, challenges exist when quizzes are placed online in LMS software. The software must be set so that students have the ability to scroll through the entire test, that is they can go back and forth to review questions. If the software is set so that students are able to see only one question at a time, the case will appear with the first question only. The student will be required to remember the nuances of the case while answering the other questions, which may result in the test assessing something it was not intended to assess—short-term memory. In addition, the test cannot be set to scramble the questions. Although this option is preferred especially when classroom testing is done in order to make cheating more difficult, scrambling the questions will separate the case from the questions that pertain to it. Scrambling the options is the only possibility.

WRITING MCQs

Test Blueprint

Test blueprints have been used in nursing education as a means to associate the number of questions on a test with the content taught and the domain and level of objectives all listed in a table format. From my perspective, the term *blueprint* is a bit of a misnomer, as only one aspect of it is completed prior to writing the questions. That aspect is knowing how many questions you plan to include on the test. However, even that decision may be delayed if questions are difficult to write or you include context-dependent questions that will take longer for students to read.

Instead of making a decision about how many questions from specific levels should be written, the focus should be on assessing the objectives. The approach that I use is to print out the blueprint table (see Exhibit 8.1) and make hash marks in each cell to indicate the number of questions that have been written for each objective at the specified level *as* I write the questions. This will avoid writing too many questions at the lower levels wof Bloom's taxonomy that are the easiest to write.

Many blueprint formats are available that include different types of information. Oermann and Gaberson (2014) and Zimmaro (2010) associated questions with specific course content, the domain and level of verb, and the number of points for each question in order to see how the exam was weighted by content. Bristol and Brett (2015) have developed fairly complex blueprints that specify the text used, NCLEX (National Council Licensure Examination) categories, QSEN (Quality and Safety Education for Nurses) competencies, the domain and level of verb, the portion of the nursing process assessed, and the question type (MCQ, fill in the blank, etc.).

The blueprint format that I have found most helpful is similar to that developed by Tarrant and Ware (2012) with the information flipped on different axes. The example of the blueprint in Exhibit 8.1 includes the levels of taxonomy (far left column), the objectives by number (second row), and the number of questions written for each objective and cognitive level (cells). A blank blueprint can also be found at www.springerpub.com/kennedy.

Choosing a specific format for the blueprint depends upon the type of information wanted and needed. The blueprint I find useful allows me to see how many questions I have developed for each objective and at what cognitive level, thus avoiding the heavy tilt toward questions from the lower

EXHIBIT 8.1
Sample Test Blueprint

Course:
Semester/Year:
Objectives:

	Cognitive Objectives					
	1	**2**	**3**	**4**	**5**	**Total**
Knowledge	1	2	1	2	1	7
Comprehension		1	2		1	4
Application	2	2	4	2	2	12
Analysis		2	2			4
Synthesis	2			2	2	6
Evaluation	2	2	1	1	1	7
Totals	7	9	10	7	7	40

Note: See the Appendix for a blank version of this template.

cognitive levels. The same type of blueprint could be created for objectives from Bloom's affective and psychomotor domains. If your course involves objectives from multiple domains, the descriptors from those domains can be added to the template in Exhibit 8.1 so a snapshot of the entire test is on one page. I would encourage you to copy/paste your objectives for the course at the top of the blueprint to maintain focus on what is to be assessed and at what level as you write the questions.

Why Question Level Matters

Because students in online nursing programs have already completed a basic nursing program and many of them have experience in clinical practice, as educators in RN to bachelor of science in nursing (BSN) and graduate nursing programs, we are in a unique position to identify misunderstandings, scaffold learning to correct them, and promote not only higher level learning, but also the development of more complex cognitive structures. Formative testing with mindfully developed MCQs that measure all aspects of Bloom's cognitive taxonomy and well-organized tests is key to achieving this. As Wiggins and McTighe (2005) summarized:

> Many students, even the best and most advanced, can *seem* to understand their work (as revealed by tests and in-class discussion) only to later reveal significant misunderstanding of what they "learned" when

follow-up questions to probe understanding are asked or application of learning is required. (pp. 51–52)

Unfortunately, research on test item banks (Masters et al., 2001) and faculty written questions (Hoseini, Shakour, Dehaghani, & Abdolmaleki, 2016; Jozefowicz et al., 2002; Vanderbilt, Feldman, & Wood, 2013; Wankhede & Kiwelekar, 2016) revealed that MCQs are often written at the lower cognitive levels of knowledge and comprehension. Unless we check for student understanding by asking higher level cognitive questions, we will never know what is understood and what is not, what is being transferred correctly and what is not. For example, when students in an introductory biology course were tested throughout the semester with higher level questions, understanding was deeper and retention longer (Jensen, McDaniel, Woodard, & Kummer, 2014).

Keep in mind that misconceptions and misunderstandings are not necessarily a failure of the educator, as students learn based on what they already know or think they know. Faculty cannot expect to understand where each student's learning begins. Consequently, development in cognitive structures can go awry and, unless we ask specific questions to assess knowledge and build additional questions to assess higher level learning, we may never know where the misunderstanding occurred. Now, realistically, this cannot be accomplished for everything we want students to understand, but doing so for the big ideas (Wiggins & McTighe, 2005) is a good place to start (see Chapter 3).

Task Analysis for Writing MCQs

MCQs must be purposely written to ensure they assess what you intend for them to assess. Thus, the desired outcome of the test you are developing should be clear in your mind before starting to write questions. If the test is formative and its purpose is for students to activate prior knowledge and review foundational content in order to prepare for the discussion, writing questions at a specific level to assess an objective is not necessary. Another purpose for a formative quiz is to make students aware of what content is important and what understandings are necessary, which will help to guide their study. Again, these questions may not assess an objective, but should be written at various levels of Bloom as is necessary for learning.

Task Analysis of an Objective

If MCQs are being written for summative assessment, which will assess one or more of the objectives, then the level of the verb used in the objective to be assessed indicates the *highest level* of question you can write. For example, if you have an objective that contains an application-level verb, it is unfair to students to write questions at the analysis, synthesis, or evaluation levels. Keep in mind that one purpose of objectives is to communicate to students what content should be learned and at which level. Thus, your test questions cannot betray that. The same is true for the other taxonomic domains. Thus, taking time to think about a task analysis pertaining to each objective is wise. This exercise will help maintain focus on the desired learning outcomes and not on the minute details of content, which is consistent with Backward Design (Wiggins & McTighe, 2005).

To illustrate how a task analysis of an objective guides the writing of test questions, we will return to the objective used in Chapter 4 for the advanced health assessment course. Both the objective and the task analysis of that objective are shown in Box 8.1. The verb *correlate* is from the synthesis level of Bloom's cognitive domain and that is what will be assessed—not only students' ability to come up with the right diagnosis, but also to demonstrate how the history guided what was assessed on the exam and how students put the pieces together to arrive at a diagnosis.

BOX 8.1
TASK ANALYSIS OF AN OBJECTIVE

Objective: *At the end of the course, the student will be able to correlate salient information from the history with abnormal findings on a focused physical examination to arrive at a plausible diagnosis.*

Component skills that must be mastered to meet this objective:

1. Ask appropriate questions on the history
2. Extract the salient data from this information
3. Based on the history, determine what systems should be assessed on exam
4. Know which basic and specialized examination techniques are indicated
5. Know how to correctly perform these basic and specialized examination techniques
6. Know what the normal findings are for the examination techniques used
7. Recognize an abnormal finding and what it indicates
8. Understand how the findings on exam validate or refute what was found on the history
9. Analyze the information to arrive at a plausible diagnosis

The results of this analysis are nine different facets of knowledge, skills, and abilities that can be used to write MCQs to assess the objective for various areas of content. Keep in mind that to fully assess this objective, more than a multiple-choice quiz may be required. For example, facet number 5 requires that faculty observe a student's performance to actually assess the objective. However, the knowledge behind the skill can be assessed with MCQs.

Identifying these facets can assist you in identifying the component knowledge and skills that are not content specific yet required to meet the objective. For each facet, questions to assess the objective can be developed from Bloom's cognitive domain, beginning at the lower levels and building to questions that will assess the objective at the appropriate level. Assessing clinical and diagnostic reasoning is inherent throughout the list. For example, the last facet indicates the result of the student's diagnostic reasoning ability. If the diagnosis is not plausible or does not logically follow from correlating findings on the history and exam, then faulty knowledge, understandings, or processes of reasoning have occurred at the level of a different facet. If questions are cognitively staged, faculty should be able to determine where the misunderstanding occurred and intervene with remediation.

Writing MCQs at Varied Cognitive Levels

A commonly heard criticism of MCQs is that they can assess only lower cognitive levels (Hoseini et al., 2016). However, Hift (2014) presented a solid argument supported by research evidence that MCQs are capable of measuring higher order cognition with the caveat that the questions must be written with this purpose in mind. This is not to minimize the need to learn facts, as they provide the foundation for higher order learning.

Cognitively Staged MCQs

Cognitively staged MCQs describe the order in which questions are delivered on a test that mimic the logical sequence of thinking that would occur when reasoning through a specific content area involved in a problem or issue. Questions that are cognitively staged begin with the lower levels of the appropriate domain and build to the level indicated by the verb in the objective. If students taking the test answer questions incorrectly, it is easy for faculty to determine misunderstandings or where their knowledge ends. This approach to testing can assist faculty in understanding the student's ZPD and intervene.

Lower cognitive level questions that do not directly assess the objective can also be used for formative assessment, whereas those written at the higher level are best suited for summative assessment, if that type of assessment is planned. However, it is important to provide practice for students in answering higher level cognitive questions during the formative assessment process in order for them to understand the full picture of how the content they are studying will be used in their chosen role.

Because questions at the lower cognitive levels of knowledge and comprehension are easier to write, that is a good place to start. These questions should focus on content that is *essential* for higher level understandings—the *must know* as opposed to the *nice to know*—that is foundational to building knowledge of the content. Next, consider how that content from the lower level questions will be applied in practice and ask the questions shown in Box 8.2.

To demonstrate what cognitively staged questions might look like and how a broadly written objective can be assessed in a specific area of content, such as hearing, let us return to the example used in the Task Analysis of an Objective section. Recall that the objective that will be assessed is, *At the end of the course, the student will be able to correlate salient information from the history with abnormal findings on a focused physical examination to arrive at a plausible diagnosis.* The verb *correlate* is from the cognitive domain, synthesis level.

The first types of questions to write are those from the levels of knowledge or comprehension. Essential knowledge related to performing the tests used to assess hearing is to know which test is the Rinne and which is the Weber. Thus, a knowledge-level MCQs might include:

1. The Weber is one of two tests done to assess hearing. The Weber is done by placing the vibrating tuning fork:
   a. On the mastoid process
   b. In front of the ear canal
   c. On the top of the head*

BOX 8.2

QUESTIONS TO ASSOCIATE CONTENT IN MCQs TO PRACTICE

1. Why is this content essential to understand?
2. How will that knowledge and understanding be used?
3. What situations will be encountered that these understandings are necessary to help problem-solve?

This question relates to the fifth facet identified in the previous section—knowing how to correctly perform basic and specialized examination techniques or the knowledge behind performance of a skill. Many other knowledge-level questions pertaining to this content can be written following the various facets.

Question 2 is a comprehension-level question and addresses the sixth facet: knowing what the normal findings are for the examination techniques used. In order to answer this question correctly, students must know which test is which, how they are performed, what the options are for results, and how to document the normal findings.

2. The results of the Weber and Rinne must be considered together to assess hearing and arrive at a diagnosis should hearing loss be present. How is normal hearing documented?
   a. Weber does not lateralize; AC = BC
   b. Weber does not lateralize; AC>BC*
   c. Weber does not lateralize; BC>AC

Following is an example of a question that combines analysis and synthesis that will assess the synthesis-level objective for this content area.

3. Mr. Smith has just returned from Hawaii, where he enjoyed surfing and swimming in the ocean for a week. Two days prior to his flight home, he developed an upper respiratory infection (URI) with the typical symptoms of runny nose, sneezing, and mild fatigue. Upon takeoff, his right ear quickly became plugged and he could not clear it. Four days later, his URI symptoms resolved and he feels generally well, but he still cannot hear out of his right ear. He is in your office for an evaluation. On exam, his right tympanic membrane is dull, slightly yellowed in color, without visible landmarks, and immobile on pneumatic otoscopy. What is your diagnosis of his right ear and what results on Weber and Rinne do you anticipate?
   a. Right serous otitis; Weber lateralizes to the right ear with BC>AC*
   b. Right serous otitis; Weber lateralizes to the left ear with AC>BC
   c. Right serous otitis; Weber does not lateralize with AC>BC

To answer this question, students must *know* the normal results for the Weber and Rinne, how they are documented, and how a normal tympanic membrane (TM) is described. They must *understand* what the findings on exam for the right TM mean from a pathophysiologic perspective when associated with the pattern of results on the Weber and Rinne. Finally, they must *analyze* information on the history that includes barotrauma associated with a URI and the findings on exam (how the TM appears and the results of the Weber and Rinne). Arriving at a diagnosis (serous otitis) that is the result of loss of the normal function of the Eustachian tube is possible by *synthesizing* (putting all of these findings together). Thus, this question addresses many of the facets of the objective mentioned earlier.

Following logically, the next question would be a synthesis question as well that asks what kind of hearing loss was demonstrated in the case, a conductive (correct answer) or sensorineural hearing loss? To answer this question, students must *know* about the two tests, Weber and Rinne, what the normal findings are when combining the results of the two tests and *understand* how the patterns differ for conductive and sensorineural hearing loss, and how each is documented. Again, they are combining information (*synthesis)* from the case to arrive at the correct type of hearing loss.

This brings up the issue as to whether asking an evaluation question may be considered unfair to students when the objective is written at the synthesis level. As arriving at a diagnosis is an expectation of an advanced health assessment course, most likely another objective will be written to cover this. So, from these questions, all levels of Bloom's cognitive domain have been addressed for this content area and two objectives partially assessed. The knowledge and comprehension questions can be used on the formative quizzes and the final two questions are appropriate for either the formative or summative quizzes. Reviewing a student's answers on these questions can be diagnostic in learning students' *understandings* (Wiggins & McTighe, 2005) of this content. As you write these questions remember to have the blueprint in front of you so you can track how many questions you are writing for each level.

The other consideration when writing cognitively staged questions is the teaching ability they have. Both formative and summative assessments using MCQs are powerful teaching tools that can exploit the testing effect as well as spaced study (Chapter 1) if students are allowed to take the test multiple times for mastery. Providing rationales for incorrect answers that students will not have access to until 24 hours after the online test has closed is another way to maximize spaced study and improve long-term retention.

Question Order on Tests

Several options exist that have research backing for the order of questions on a test. Questions can be organized by:

- Test item format so that similar formats are grouped together, that is, all MCQs are listed first, followed by true–false, matching, context-dependent sets, and so forth

- Order of item difficulty, starting with the easier questions to allay student anxiety
- The order of how the content was taught in the course
- By type of content, that is, questions on similar content are grouped together, such as all content on the renal system followed by that on the cardiac system

Although all methods of ordering items on a test are used in nursing, choosing the order often seems a bit arbitrary, and not evidence based. In a meta-analysis, Aamodt and McShane (1992) studied the ordering of questions on tests and found that organizing test questions from easy to difficult did not significantly improve test scores over random ordering, but produced notably less anxiety, which for weaker students could affect confidence and potentially their performance. Conversely, starting an exam with more difficult items compared to using random order significantly decreased exam scores. Exams ordered by content showed no difference in performance over random ordering.

Test item order may also affect the way in which students perceive their performance. Weinstein and Roediger (2012) found that students were more likely to overestimate their performance when questions were ordered from easy to hard as compared to sorting from hard to easy or in random order. This post-test-taking bias may result in more e-mails or phone calls to faculty asking if the test was accurately scored. However, research is not aligned in this respect, as a study by Vander Schee (2013) found no difference in performance on an exam related to test item order. To offset students' post-test-taking global impressions, Weinstein and Roediger (2012) conducted a study in which two groups of students took the same 100-item test containing the same questions in a different order. The questions in the test for one group were ordered from easy to hard, and the opposite order used in the other group. Students in both groups were stopped after every 10 questions to ask their impressions of their performance, to query their overall impression of the test, and to predict their final grade. The results indicated that students felt more optimistic about their performance when questions were ordered from easy to hard even though actual performance was equal. However, they were more sensitive to questions becoming more difficult as the test progressed.

Until more consistent research findings come to light, I would recommend starting a quiz with a few easier questions to decrease anxiety and increase confidence and then proceed with questions in a random order. However, if you are using cognitively staged questions, you may want to order them in a logical order from simple to complex following the taxonomy being used.

Logistical Considerations

Formative Assessment Online

Providing a multiple-choice quiz as a formative assessment with each module and allowing students to take it multiple times for mastery maximizes the testing effect and spaced study and will strengthen retrieval cues that will subsequently improve long-term memory and promote transfer (Roediger & Karpicke, 2006). The most appropriate type of question for our students may be the MCQ, as the format is consistent with the type students will encounter on certification boards. In terms of the timing of these quizzes, students should initially take this quiz prior to studying the content to retrieve prior knowledge in order to understand what they know and do not know, which will subsequently guide their study. Based on the research, at least 1 day of no study should follow the study session before taking the test the second time. This is not something faculty can control, but in the introduction to the first module, sharing research findings from cognitive science on spaced study (Chapter 1) with students may help them realize the benefits of the approach you are suggesting.

If the questions include the correct answer and two distractors, conceivably three opportunities to take the quiz could be allowed. However, with three opportunities comes the chance for students to zip through the test using the process of elimination in a rote fashion, guessing at the answers. By the third try, they will have answered all questions correctly without having learned anything at all. So, my advice is to give students one less try than the number of options. So, for questions with three options, they should be given two opportunities to take the quiz.

Feedback should be provided on the distractors (incorrect answers) without providing the correct answer, but instead guiding remedial study. Feedback in the form of where the content can be found in their text, a link to a website or journal article, or a metacognitive or probing question to guide their thinking are all forms of useful feedback in a constructivist paradigm.

If three attempts are allowed on a quiz, the first time being prior to studying, I recommend that the grades on the second and third opportunities be averaged for the actual quiz grade. This will encourage taking the quizzes seriously and discourage guessing. Ideally, students should be able to review their answers on these quizzes prior to the midterm or final, should faculty feel these summative tests are necessary.

Formative or Summative?

The question arises as to whether these quizzes to promote learning are formative or summative. By definition, they are formative in that they are tests to *promote* learning or test *for* learning. However, we all know that students rarely complete activities that are optional and do not carry a point value. Consequently, a few points should be attached to each quiz. Keep in mind that these tests do not assess learning or mastery of the content even though points are earned. Thus, they should not be considered assessment *of* learning. This is a distinction I would make when providing instructions on the quizzes for students so they are in the right frame of mind when they take them.

If summative tests are the main type of assessment used in your online course, there are a few things to keep in mind. First, even though you tell students it is a closed-book test, you can never be assured that they will comply. Second, you can only assume that they are the one taking the test, and they are doing so alone without the help of others. Third, online tests can be copied and pasted to a Word document and shared with future classes. Obviously, shared tests no longer have much value as summative assessments. Although these are all violations of the honor code and are considered academic dishonesty, some students will push the envelope. This must be taken into consideration when planning an online, high-stakes test that will have an impact on final grades.

LMSs include features to help you dissuade students from cheating. Timing the test and allowing several minutes for each question often keeps students from looking up answers in their textbooks. However, if you include many case-based questions that take time to read, more time should be allotted per question. Another way to steer students away from their texts is to write questions whose answers cannot be found in their readings. Limit the number of knowledge- and comprehension-level questions, and instead write questions at the application level and above in the cognitive domain for which foundational knowledge is necessary to answer them.

Students sharing answers with a classmate is a concern in online testing. If you have written conventional-format questions, you can shuffle the questions so that each student basically has a different test—questions are randomly ordered. If you are using cases with multiple questions referring to one case, then shuffling the questions themselves is not an option. The questions will become separated from the case. You can shuffle the options (correct answer and distractors) so that the answer to the first question will be "a" for one student, for example, and "c" for another.

Some LMSs have a lock system that once activated will not allow students to surf the Internet. Although this is useful when students take a test on campus in a computer lab or in a classroom using their laptops, it is not effective for remote online testing. Students can search the net on their smartphone or tablet, so blocking that function on their computer has little meaning and often causes technology issues as students struggle to set it up on their computers.

Do prepare students for the type of questions on a summative assessment by including similar questions on the formative tests. Often, you can reword questions to use on both tests. Remember that your goal is to assess what they learned as applied to their future role, not the minutiae of what was taught.

THE TAKE-AWAY

Multiple-choice tests have a place in nursing education as both formative and summative assessments and methods of reinforcing content. Frequent formative MCQ assessments take full advantage of the testing effect to improve retrieval and long-term retention and are easy to make available to students in the online environment. Summative tests are problematic online as faculty members have little control over the test-taking environment and must rely on students' integrity. Even if MCQs can be written at higher levels of the various taxonomies, more appropriate types of summative assessment exist, such as online question- or case-based discussions. However, questions purposely written at various levels of the taxonomies to promote learning and potentially assess the objectives will help students build rich mental models, allow faculty to determine students' ZPD, scaffold learning when needed, and help them be successful in their future role.

REFERENCES

Aamodt, M. G., & McShane, T. (1992). A meta-analytic investigation of the effect of various test item characteristics on test scores. *Public Personnel Management, 21,* 151–160.

Bristol, T., & Brett, A. L. (2015). Test item writing: 3Cs for successful tests. *Teaching and Learning in Nursing, 10,* 100–103.

Carpenter, S. K. (2012). Testing enhances the transfer of learning. *Current Directions in Psychological Science, 21*(5), 279–283.

Haladyna, T. M. (2004). *Developing and validating multiple-choice test items.* Mahwah, NJ: Lawrence Erlbaum.

Haladyna, T. M., & Downing, S. M. (1993). How many options is enough for a multiple-choice test item? *Educational and Psychological Measurement, 54,* 999–1010.

Hift, R. J. (2014). Should essays and other open-ended-type questions retain a place in written summative assessment in clinical medicine? *BMC Medical Education, 14*(1). Retrieved from http://www.biomedcentral.com/1472-6920/14/249

Hoseini, H., Shakour, M., Dehaghani, A. R., & Abdolmaleki, M. R. (2016). An investigation of various quality indicators of final exams in specialized courses of

Bachelor of Nursing. *International Journal of Educational and Psychological Researches*, 2(1), 60–64.

Jensen, J. L., McDaniel, M. A., Woodard, S. M., & Kummer, T. A. (2014). Teaching to the test . . . or testing to teach: Exams requiring higher order thinking skills encourage greater conceptual understanding. *Educational Psychology Review*, 26(2), 307–329.

Jozefowicz, R. F., Koeppen, B. M., Case, S., Galbraith, R., Swanson, D., & Glew, R. H. (2002). The quality of in-house medical school examinations. *Academic Medicine*, 77(2), 156–161.

Kilgour, J. M., & Tayyaba, S. (2015). An investigation into the optimal number of distractors in single-best answer exams. *Advances in Health Science Education*, 21(3), 1–15. Retrieved from http://link.springer.com/article/10.1007/s10459-015-9652-7

Masters, J. C., Hulsmeyer, B. S., Pike, M. E., Leichty, K., Miller, M. T., & Verst, A. L. (2001). Assessment of multiple-choice questions in selected test banks accompanying textbooks used in nursing education. *Journal of Nursing Education*, 40(1), 25–32.

Mayer, R. E. (1998). Cognitive, metacognitive, and motivational aspects of problem solving. *Instructional Science*, 26, 49–63.

Merriam, S. B., & Leahy, B. (2005). Learning transfer: A review of the research in adult education and training. *PAACE Journal of Lifelong Learning*, 14, 1–24.

Oermann, M. H., & Gaberson, K. B. (2014). *Evaluation and testing in nursing education*. New York, NY: Springer Publishing.

Rodriguez, M. C. (2005). Three options are optimal for multiple-choice items: A meta-analysis of 80 years of research. *Educational Measurement: Issues and Practice*, 24(2), 3–13.

Roediger, H. L., & Karpicke, J. D. (2006). The power of testing memory: Basic research and implications for educational practice. *Perspectives on Psychological Science*, 1(3), 181–210.

Schneid, S. D., Armour, C., Park, Y. S., Yudkowsky, R., & Bordage, G. (2014). Reducing the number of options on multiple-choice questions: Response time, psychometrics and standard setting. *Medical Education*, 48(10), 1020–1027.

Tarrant, M., & Ware, J. (2012). A framework for improving the quality of multiple-choice assessments. *Nurse Educator*, 37(3), 98–104.

Vanderbilt, A. A., Feldman, M., & Wood, I. K. (2013). Assessment in undergraduate medical education: A review of course exams. *Medical Education Online, 18*. Retrieved from http://www.ncbi.nlm.nih.gov/pmc/articles/PMC3591508/pdf/MEO-18-20438.pdf

Vander Schee, B. A. (2013). Test item order, level of difficulty, and student performance in marketing education. *Journal of Education for Business*, 88, 36–42.

Wankhede, H. S., & Kiwelekar, A. W. (2016). Qualitative assessment of software engineering examination questions with Bloom's taxonomy. *Indian Journal of Science and Technology*, 9(6). Retrieved from http://www.indjst.org/index.php/indjst/article/view/85012

Weinstein, Y., & Roediger, H. L., III. (2012). The effect of question order on evaluations of test performance: How does the bias evolve? *Memory & Cognition*, 40, 727–735.

Wiggins, G., & McTighe, J. (2005). *Understanding by design* (2nd ed.). Alexandria, VA: Association for Supervision and Curriculum Development.
Zimmaro, D. M. (2010). *Writing good multiple-choice exams.* Austin, TX: Center for Teaching and Learning, University of Texas at Austin. Retrieved from https://facultyinnovate.utexas.edu/sites/default/files/documents/Writing-Good-Multiple-Choice-Exams-04-28-10.pdf

9

Grading and the Rubric

Although rubrics are used almost exclusively in higher education as grading schemes for summative assessment (Reddy & Andrade, 2010), their use in formative assessment is explored in this chapter. How did we get here? Why use rubrics to assess performance? A brief review of grading practices in higher education may help shed light on why the need for greater objectivity in grading has gained increasing attention and how a well-structured rubric can fill the bill.

GRADING IN HIGHER EDUCATION

Grading is probably one of the most important tasks, the most time consuming, and the least desirable for faculty. Countless hours can be spent in grading discussion boards and written assignments—providing feedback that students often ignore—for it is the grade itself that receives the most attention. Grades have implications and consequences for a variety of stakeholders and often form the basis for gatekeeping administrative decisions, such as academic progression within a degree program, admission for an advanced degree, suitability for scholarships and academic honors, and program accreditation, not to mention the effect on student self-esteem, learning, and persistence (Sadler, 2010). Thus, the responsibility inherent in grading is heavy. Judgments on student work must be made ethically, objectively, and from a defensible position. Milligan (1996) offered some sound advice. When referring to grading student work, he feels it should be done based on clearly written and well-understood criteria.

> If such clarification [of the grading criteria] is not given or the punitive weapon of unsubstantiated professional judgment is the only, or most important criteria [sic] used, then the asessor [sic] is possibly left with litle [sic] credibility and fails to meet the standard stated here of acting ethically in assessment matters. (p. 414)

This perspective is related to what Sadler (2010) referred to as *fidelity* in grading or "the extent to which elements that contribute to a course grade are correctly identified as academic achievement" (p. 728). This is an important point and one that is easy to lose sight of because of personal beliefs held by faculty and specific grading practices at the school or university. Grade inflation, which is so rampant in higher education, has overshadowed the concept of fidelity in grading (Scanlan & Care, 2004). However, when developing criteria for grading, faculty must be clear on how the objectives have defined academic achievement for the course.

GRADING AND ACADEMIC ACHIEVEMENT

According to Sadler (2010), *achievement* was defined as "the attainment of an identifiable level of knowledge or skill as determined through evaluating performances on assessment tasks, or through observation of relevant behaviours in specified settings" (p. 730). Grades are the overt measurement of academic achievement that are made explicit to students and shared with other stakeholders. Do they reflect true academic achievement or something else?

Course Components Not Related to Academic Achievement

Sadler's (2010) definition of fidelity encouraged faculty to be sure that grades reflect true academic achievement that is defined by the course objectives. Courses and learning should be outcome focused with the objectives driving what is assessed, and assessing the objectives should represent what students have learned. If a downside exists to broadly written objectives, it is that they do not provide sufficient detail for meaningful grading of assignments, so assessment criteria must be written for everything that you will grade. However, as is current practice, other variables are often included in students' course grades, which Sadler refers to as transactional, bestowed, and regulative credits and debits that are not related to academic achievement.

Transactional credits refer to points awarded for attendance, participation alone, and completion of activities such as journal entries or preliminary drafts of a final paper. *Transactional debits* are points deducted for turning in assignments late or for plagiarism (Sadler, 2010).

Bestowed credits are those "awarded entirely at the assessor's discretion" (Sadler, 2010, p. 732) and are sometimes done unconsciously, I would add, when giving the student *the benefit of the doubt*. This type of credit includes rewarding students with points *for effort* put into an assignment, obvious performance improvement over time, thinking outside the box, and to compensate for a student's illness or other personal emergency. Bestowed credits involve adjusting points for an assignment that faculty felt was poorly explained, or to compensate for students at a perceived disadvantage (e.g., for whom English is not their primary language). This type of credit is often given to avoid failing a student or placing him or her in jeopardy of losing a scholarship. Some faculty want to avoid upsetting the student—or having to deal with an upset student may be more accurate—so points are not deducted when they should have been. This often engenders "good feelings" on the part of the student toward the faculty member that are reflected in the end-of-course student surveys that can have an impact on faculty retention and promotion.

Points are often awarded or deducted for what Sadler (2010) terms *regulative* issues, which really relate to *compliance,* in my view, and that are often spelled out in the instructions for each assignment or within the rubric. Assignment requirements, such as the specific word count, required number of references, and adherence to a specific writing and format style such as the American Psychological Association (APA), are often awarded points, but most likely are not elements included in the course objectives. Although mastery of APA format and development of a professional writing style are desired programmatic outcomes, if these competencies or outcomes are not included in the course objectives, then they cannot be included as part of a final grade or considered as part of academic achievement. Yet, time spent grading papers often focuses on writing style and APA format at the expense of comments on content and flow of ideas.

Probably the main area where faculty spend inordinate amounts of time, in my opinion, is editing student papers . . . not providing formative feedback, but actually making corrections on syntax, grammar, and writing style using track changes in Word in courses where writing is not the focus, nor are these skills included in the objectives. And, when track changes are used, all the student has to do is "accept all changes" and the document is "where faculty wants it." This practice does not support learning from a constructivist perspective.

However, faculty have two options. One option is to provide formative feedback on writing style and format without point benefit or penalty, hoping the student will learn from the feedback and improve on the next assignment. The other option is to return the assignment to the student for revision based on *true* formative feedback that points out the errors by asking questions, such as "Is that the correct reference format for a journal article?" or "Did you omit some information in the in-text citation?" A grade is then withheld on the assignment until these errors are corrected. In this regard, faculty are not actually correcting the mistakes, but giving the student the opportunity to do so and learn in the process. In my view, the second option is a sound constructivist practice, as it is the student doing the work and not faculty. It will also result in deeper learning. However, unless there is oversight across courses and some type of program-driven, top-down accountability for achieving programmatic goals, students may continue to make the same errors and not be held accountable to learn.

ACADEMIC ACHIEVEMENT AND COURSE OBJECTIVES

Decisions as to what will be assessed should be made based on the course objectives and with the concepts of fidelity and the measurement of academic achievement in mind. Elements that do *not* represent mastery of course outcomes, but are commonly included in the final course grade, are:

- Posting in a discussion for the purpose of meeting the requirement for initial course attendance
- Nonsubstantive contributions to discussion boards, such as posts that do not contribute to the discourse in a meaningful way
- Completion of reflective journals in which an outcome is not specified in the objectives, or reflection on course content not required in the journal entries
- Completion of sections of a larger assignment that will be again graded when completed. If the sections and total assignment are graded, the work is graded twice, thus doubling the actual percentage the assignment contributes to the final grade
- Conforming to elements of assignments that are considered requirements, such as adhering to the maximum number of words in a discussion post or assignment, or proper APA formatting for in-text citations and references unless included in the course objectives

How faculty choose to assess the objectives for the course determines how academic achievement is defined, and a certain amount of academic freedom goes into making this decision. However, the decision should be made with a solid understanding of grading fidelity. Perhaps putting this decision in a different context will help. What can occur if faculty do not fully understand the ramifications of translating course outcomes indicated by the objectives to points could make the difference in a student who has really not met the learning outcomes passing a course.

So, what are the options? Providing formative feedback without adding a point value so that students know how to improve sections of a paper prior to the final submission is good practice. The rubric for the assignment can serve as the basis for this type of formative assessment without points being recorded as part of the process. However, what will most likely grab students' attention and get them to use the feedback on all sections is seeing an actual grade. In this case, faculty could overcome this by including a *potential* grade, that is, giving students an idea of what the grade would be at each juncture.

Most of the writing-related issues can be dealt with at the program level by mapping the curriculum to identify courses in which writing will be an outcome and adding the appropriately worded objectives so that this skill is assessed. When writing is an outcome assigned to specific courses, I recommend that sections of the assignment be turned in at regular intervals during the semester, formative feedback be provided for each section, and that a lesser point value then be assigned to the final iteration of the paper as it represents your feedback incorporated into the student's work. This approach will ensure that students make their best effort writing each section, that any misunderstanding or misinterpretation of the assignment criteria does not occur, and that students have the opportunity to create a polished version as a final representation of what they learned in the course. From the faculty's perspective, if students pay attention to the feedback, the final paper should be relatively easy to grade.

The final paper, including all segments turned in (with faculty comments), should then be uploaded to each student's e-portfolio, and that portfolio made available to all faculty in the program who will teach courses where writing is an identified outcome. This approach has several advantages. First, students will understand the value placed on writing skills and be hard-pressed to ignore feedback, as points will be deducted if the outcomes are not met. In addition, they will know that their work, including faculty feedback, will follow them throughout the program, eliminating the impact of comments such as "I didn't know" or "I was never told" when referring to faculty feedback. This will also encourage faculty to know APA format well, so that consistent feedback is given. Second, this approach offers faculty the option and ability to refer to previously graded papers to determine if students are correcting their errors based on feedback. If not, this should be called to the student's attention early on and an action plan developed. Providing the same comments over and over takes a great deal of faculty time and is not productive if the student is not paying attention.

Third, when writing outcomes are reflected in the objectives, meeting the objectives becomes a competency issue. In the courses where writing skills are assessed, faculty should take the time to review how the student has progressed in this regard by taking a look at the papers most recently uploaded to the e-portfolio. If assessment of the papers has been done using an iterative approach (discussed in Chapter 6) and faculty have been diligent in providing formative feedback throughout the program, students' writing skills should be progressing. From the outset of their program, how writing skills will be assessed, in which courses, and the point allocation for each writing assignment with any point penalties for late or missed submissions should be clearly explained and a handout provided and included in the student handbook.

This approach will ensure that writing is a program competency that students will be supported in meeting. It will also avoid faculty spending undue amounts of time providing feedback on writing skills in courses where writing is not a specified outcome. The question of defining academic achievement will also be addressed, helping faculty to focus on assessing the actual learning outcomes.

Assessment of writing and APA formatting skills applies to discussion board posts as well. Discussions are the hallmark of online teaching and assessment, but, again, unless these skills are included in the course objectives, they are not considered elements of academic achievement.

Finally, faculty awareness of the issues surrounding the assessment of true academic achievement is paramount. Simply considering grade integrity, fidelity, and the dichotomy of what constitutes academic achievement and what does not will set the stage for identifying appropriate performance criteria for rubrics and appropriate grading. In the end, most likely other creative strategies to combat the age-old argument that *if students aren't graded on an activity, they will not do it* may need to be developed, but done so keeping grade integrity and the assessment of actual academic achievement in mind.

RUBRIC OVERVIEW

Rubrics are grading tools that specify multiple levels of performance, ranging from beginning or novice level to that most desired or competent, and include a scoring strategy for each level. Two types of rubrics have been used in higher education, the holistic rubric and the analytic rubric, also called a *grading rubric*. The holistic rubric assesses work more globally and is used most often for writing assignments. In this type of rubric, multiple criteria are listed under a single scoring strategy (Mertler, 2001). For example, various levels of performance might be included for grammar, punctuation, sentence structure, and so on. Exhibit 9.1 depicts the typical format for a holistic rubric in which the levels of performance for the ideal score are at the top of the rubric and the lowest score, perhaps those characteristics associated with zero points, are at the bottom. The lower levels are not shown here. This rubric is rarely used in higher education because of the inherent difficulties of students adequately meeting all criteria associated with one score. The analytic rubric, the focus of the remainder of this chapter, is used more often as its design is better suited to individualized, specific, and objective feedback.

EXHIBIT 9.1
Holistic Rubric Format

5—Consistently does the following
• Does not misspell any words
• Uses proper syntax
• No grammatical errors
• In-text citations are in proper APA format
• References are in proper APA format
4—Does many of the following
• Occasionally misspells words
• Occasionally uses improper syntax
• Occasionally makes a grammatical error
• Occasionally uses incorrect in-text APA citation format
• Occasionally uses incorrect APA reference format
3—Rarely does any of the following

APA, American Psychological Association.

Purpose of a Rubric

The purpose of a rubric is to increase objectivity and ideally intra- and interrater reliability in grading (Newell, Dahm, & Newell, 2002). A rubric that clearly spells out the ideal performance is beneficial for both faculty and students. For faculty, detailed feedback is innate within the rubric eliminating the need to write the same comments again and again (Isaacson & Stacy, 2009), making the grading process more efficient. The benefit for students is that assignment expectations are made explicit. When assessment rubrics are disseminated with the course syllabus as the semester begins, students have a clear understanding of expected performance and can use the rubric as a checklist for assignment components (Popham, 1997).

Rubrics can be used for both formative and summative assessments. Because awarding points is associated with summative assessment, rubrics are most often used for that purpose. Recall from Chapter 1 that formative assessment, or assessment *for* learning, involves providing feedback to students to indicate what they have done well and where improvement is needed, which is typically done while the assignment is in progress before a grade is assigned. Iterative grading, a type of formative assessment that allows students to revise and resubmit their work to incorporate the feedback, is an excellent approach to promote deep learning, although repeated review is time consuming for faculty (Gikandi, Morrowa, & Davis, 2011; Jonsson, 2013). Rubrics can be used for formative assessment without recording the grade, but an explanation to students is warranted. Explain that the purpose of demonstrating to them the points they would have earned on the assignment, should a grade be given at that juncture, will often drive the message home in a way meaningful to extrinsically motivated students.

Summative assessment, or assessment *of* learning, involves assigning a numerical grade or pass/fail status (Kennedy, Chan, Fok, & Yu, 2008). This typically signals the end of the conversation on the assignment, although students have been known to challenge their grades.

The point of reviewing formative and summative assessment is to underscore their relationship to fidelity and academic achievement. Becoming clear on how you are defining academic achievement for the course and what will be assessed are decisions you must make early on during the course-planning phase. Formative and summative assessment on discussions and assignments must be the same for each assignment. Obviously, you cannot have one set of criteria that is used to provide formative feedback and another for summative assessment. Students will not understand *what you want*—a common concern often voiced when outcomes are not clearly articulated. Nevertheless, rubrics can be used to provide formative feedback without points being allocated, so the criteria should be the same for both.

THE ANALYTIC RUBRIC

Popham's (1997) original description of analytic or grading rubrics remains the standard today. An analytic rubric by definition has three elements that distinguish it from other types of grading tools and is displayed in a grid-like format. These three elements are listed in Box 9.1.

Defining these terms, providing examples of each, and viewing an example of this type of rubric will help to visualize the analytic rubric format. As the descriptive names of these elements can be confusing, referring to Exhibit 9.2 will help the reader understand their placement in the template.

BOX 9.1
ELEMENTS OF AN ANALYTIC RUBRIC

1. *Performance criteria* (titles in far left column)
2. *Performance descriptors* explain the expectations of each assessment criterion along a continuum from beginning level to ideal performance for each category (in rows)
3. A *scoring strategy* (column heading) signifies the points associated with each level of performance for each criterion (for each cell)

EXHIBIT 9.2
Analytic Rubric Format

Performance Criteria	Beginning performance 2 points	Intermediate performance 3 points	Ideal performance 4 points	Total points
Criterion 1	Performance descriptor Criterion 1	Performance descriptor Criterion 1	Performance descriptor Criterion 1	
Criterion 2	Performance descriptor Criterion 2			
Criterion 3	Performance descriptor Criterion 3			
Criterion 4	Performance descriptor Criterion 4			
Criterion 5	Performance descriptor Criterion 5			
			Earned percentage	
			Potential points for assignment	
			Earned points	

Performance Criteria

Placed in the far left column of the rubric, performance criteria are titles indicating *categories* that summarize the performance to be evaluated. Often omitted from rubrics (Dawson, 2015), they act as labels and provide visual organization for the reader. In addition, when a rubric assesses complex tasks, it is often necessary to divide these categories into multiple subcategories, making these labels even more important for organization.

Controversy exists over the ideal number of performance criteria, which can vary with the performance being assessed and the level of granularity desired. Popham (1997) recommends limiting the number of performance categories to five. For example, in creating a rubric to assess nurse practitioner students' written SOAP (subjective, objective, assessment, plan) note for an advanced health assessment course, these criteria might be, "history," "exam," "assessment," and "overall note," referring to how well the student connected the various categories in the assignment through critical thinking or diagnostic reasoning. An additional benefit of including these titles is that they provide clarity on the specific construct being evaluated as faculty write the performance descriptions so the intent remains true.

Performance Descriptors

Once the performance criteria have been identified, the next step is to write descriptions for the various levels of performance that are each associated with a different score. Writing these descriptions is the most challenging and important aspect of rubric development. *Performance descriptors* are concise phrases (not complete sentences) that specify and distinguish observable levels of performance on a continuum for each performance criterion. As shown in Exhibit 9.2, the descriptions of performance are placed in rows starting with the beginning level of performance on the left and progressing to the desired performance on the right, a natural progression or continuum.

The goal when writing these descriptors is to develop clear and mutually exclusive language for each level of performance, as each description is associated with a separate scoring strategy. While this can be challenging, it can be accomplished if a few guidelines are followed. These include maintaining focus on a single construct for each criterion, varying the quality or quantity of performance for each instead of using different verbiage, and using language that describes the performance as opposed to judging it. This assures that there is reliability of interpretation for both students and faculty (Moskal, 2000) and no subjective decisions must be made. In order for the rubric to meet the dual goals of being objective and promoting interrater reliability, faculty should not have difficulty deciding between levels of performance when using the rubric as a grading tool. In other words, performance descriptors should not overlap and should include only one concept or construct. Maintaining focus as you write the descriptions for the various levels can be accomplished by referring to the performance criterion or title. Thus, deciding on a descriptive title is crucial.

Deciding on the number of levels of performance is essential to developing a useful rubric and goes hand in hand with what can be realistically written without overlap. However, controversy exists regarding the optimal number of levels. Bresciani, Zelna, and Anderson (2004) advocated only three levels of performance, citing difficulties for students in absorbing the multiple levels toward mastery as well as for faculty in creating mutually exclusive descriptions. Mertler (2001) recommended four descriptors. However, I tend to agree with Moskal (2000) in that it is better to have a few meaningful and easily understood descriptors rather than many that overlap, resulting in a cumbersome rubric that is impossible for students to use when completing the assignment and equally challenging for faculty when grading. Thus, the number of descriptors for each criterion really depends on the number of meaningful levels of performance that can be written while maintaining the uniqueness of each.

Perhaps the easiest way to determine the number of performance levels is to actually write them. Mertler (2001) recommended developing the verbiage for the ideal performance first, and I must agree that this is the best approach. Once the desired performance has been clearly described, Moskal (2000) advocated turning attention to the *lowest* level, which can be approached by considering common mistakes students make on this particular performance. These are the comments faculty find themselves writing repeatedly when they grade the assignment that can become the foundation for not only the lowest level, but also the other levels of performance (Isaacson & Stacy, 2009). Next, write a level in between. If an additional level can be written and remain unique, you have determined the number of levels of performance for each criterion. Remember that all performance criteria should have the same number of levels if possible. Occasionally, performance is either present or not present, in which case a line can be drawn through the other levels, in order to indicate to faculty and students that this performance is dichotomous.

An example of how levels of performance can be written may help to clarify this important step. Returning to the previous SOAP note example, a difficult concept for students to grasp is which elements from the review of systems (ROS) should be included in a brief, focused note. Their choices often seem to be random and do not enlighten the chief complaint. The performance description for the lowest level criterion might include that common mistake and read: *ROS includes random elements that do not pertain to the chief complaint.* Appropriate language for the mid-level criterion might be: *ROS includes some pertinent elements that pertain to the chief complaint.* The ideal performance might state: *ROS includes* only *pertinent elements from ROS that pertain to the chief complaint.* Comparing these three levels of performance, students understand what they need to do to perform well and earn all points. This underscores instruction and reminds students that the reader of a SOAP note should be able to delimit the chief complaint and understand what is being ruled out based on the history alone.

In some instances, levels of performance can be specified quantitatively using *includes 25% of the variable* with the subsequent levels being 50% and 90%. A perfect 100% may not be a realistic goal for students, so exercise caution when using this marker as the ideal level of performance. Alternatively, the number of items to be included in each performance level can be specified, such as *includes zero to one* element of the performance, *includes two to three,* and for the desired performance, *includes at least three,* again with the understanding that three elements does not indicate 100%. These various approaches will help to avoid the pitfall of adding new concepts or constructs to the descriptors as they are being developed, a common mistake.

A word of caution is in order here. Avoid using a progression such as rarely, usually, and always for a rubric meant to grade one assessment, as this progression suggests a comparison of assessments over time. For example, consider this wording for the beginning level of performance: *Rarely includes all pertinent elements of the cardiac exam in the SOAP note.* This wording does not seem to indicate how the student has done on the note being graded, but that his or her performance has consistently not been up to par.

Including more than one construct in each level of performance creates a dilemma when the student performs well on one and not on the other, requiring faculty to make a subjective decision as to what score to assign and causing interrater reliability to suffer. For example, I have often encountered a descriptor of the ideal level of writing performance that reads: *Writing style is professional and references and citations are in correct APA format.* The grading dilemma occurs if the student's writing style is professional, he or she has made frequent errors in APA formatting of the references, and the in-text citations are well done. Clearly, writing style and APA format are two separate constructs that, if a desired outcome is reflected in the objectives, deserve to be in separate criteria.

Descriptors should include language that actually describes the performance being assessed and not a judgment about that performance (Moskal, 2000). Returning to the SOAP note example to explain this idea, a description of how the ROS was incorporated into the note on the lowest performance level might read: *ROS includes random elements that do not pertain to the chief complaint.* Contrast these with the following, which indicates a judgment about this specific performance: *ROS is poorly done.* This wording is inadequate in terms of providing guidance to students when completing the assignment, and does not give specific direction on how to improve their work when the rubric is used to provide formative feedback.

Remember that all performance criteria should have the same number of levels of performance, if possible. Occasionally, performance is dichotomous, either present or not, in which case a line can be drawn through the other levels of performance where a descriptor should be used to indicate to faculty and students that only two choices exist.

In summary, writing concise and understandable performance descriptors can be achieved by following a few recommendations: (a) avoid overlap in the descriptions of performance as they progress from beginner to desired performance; (b) include the same construct in all performance descriptors along the continuum, varying in degree or level of performance; and (c) limit each performance descriptor to one concept/construct.

Scoring Strategy

The scoring strategy is the final element of the rubric to be considered. Analytic rubrics typically include numerical ratings that head the columns containing the performance descriptors for each criterion (see Exhibit 9.2). A common complaint heard from students is that they do not understand how points were allocated, what they must do to improve, and why they earned the grade they did. For these reasons as well as decreasing choices for faculty and improving interrater reliability, each column should contain *one* score and not a range of scores.

In addition to a numerical score, each column may also include a descriptor, such as *accomplished novice, advanced beginner,* and *competent,* which incorporates Benner's (1984/2001) early stages of professional development, adds meaning for the nursing student, and further underscores that mastery of performance occurs along a continuum. When considering verbiage to use for these descriptors, look to the program and educational level of the students. For example, *accomplished novice, advanced beginner,* and *competent* might be appropriate for the doctor of nursing practice (DNP) student who has some experience as a nurse. A label of *novice* might be insulting. Also, it is unlikely that students will graduate from a DNP program as experts, so assigning that level of Benner's continuum would be inappropriate and potentially cause undue stress. For the PhD program, descriptors such as *emerging, developing, proficient,* and *exemplary* may be consistent with program goals (Wu, Heng, & Wang, 2015).

Allen and Tanner (2006) advocated four levels of performance and recommend four labeling strategies, two of which are (a) *beginning, developing, accomplished,* and *exemplary;* or (b) *unacceptable, acceptable, proficient,* and *exemplary.* Moskal (2003) and Mertler (2001) advised choosing words that describe the quality of the work and avoid judgmental terms such as *good, better,* and *best.* Others (Newell et al., 2002) suggest that perhaps the best approach is to use numbers exclusively, citing difficulties with faculty becoming distracted with qualitative descriptions such as *excellent, very good, good,* instead of focusing on the actual descriptions of performance.

I disagree with one aspect of the overall organization of the rubric in general and the scoring strategy specifically that is seen in most published articles on rubrics (Allen & Tanner, 2006; Isaacson & Stacey, 2009; Lunney & Sammarco, 2009; Reddy & Andrade, 2010; Truemper, 2004) that has to do with how the scoring strategy is placed. It seems counterintuitive to place the ideal performance in the first column and the lowest level in the last performance column. Consequently, I place the ideal performance on the right in the column next to the column totals.

As the assignment is graded, the scores corresponding with the student's performance for each of the performance criteria (cell ratings) are summed to arrive at a total score, which is then listed in the far right column on the rubric. Unless the total score computed from this method equals the actual point value for the assignment, which is difficult to do, faculty must first calculate the percentage score. This is accomplished by dividing the student's earned points by the number of points that would indicate a perfect score based on the rubric. For example, if the highest scoring strategy was four points and six performance criteria were included in the rubric, the maximum score attainable would be 24 points. Thus, if the student earned 20 out of 24 possible points, the percentage earned is 83%. If the assignment was worth 15 points, another calculation would be required to arrive at the actual points earned.

I found this method not only cumbersome, but also recognized that the inherent assumption is that all performance criteria were considered to be of equal weight. For example, when grading a SOAP note in an advanced health assessment course, the skill to be mastered is writing a succinct yet inclusive history that paints an accurate picture of the patient, which logically results in a correct diagnosis or differential diagnoses. Recall that the performance categories were history, exam, assessment, and overall note. The final criterion reflected the student's critical thinking and diagnostic reasoning ability and became more important as learning progressed through the semester than in the first SOAP note assignment. For the first few SOAP note assignments, the history and exam portions of the note deserved a heavier weighting as part of the learning curve in writing a succinct note. Toward the end of the semester more weight should be placed on the overall note criterion, reflecting the ability to integrate the elements of the note to arrive at a diagnosis. The ability to weight performance criteria allows faculty to use the same rubric to grade all similar assignments for a course by adjusting the weighting for each criterion as appropriate. This approach would work well, for example, when segments of a final assignment were turned in throughout the semester.

Weighting of Criteria

However, the standard rubric scoring strategy does not provide the flexibility to weight the performance criteria; all criteria are automatically equally weighted. This prompted me to develop a scoring strategy that weights each performance criteria, and is based on a total score of 100, which then automatically becomes a percentage. Multiplied by the point value of the assignment, the product becomes the actual points students have earned on the assignment. Although other authors (Bradshaw & Lowenstein, 2011) have recognized the value in weighting performance criteria, the strategy they employed did not simplify the math.

With the goal of weighting the performance criteria and improving efficiency when grading, each performance criterion is assigned a point value or weight (see the second column labeled "criterion value" in Exhibit 9.3. In order for the final score to become a percentage, the product of rows multiplied by columns must equal 100 for the ideal or perfect performance. Consequently, the sum of the criterion value column must be adjusted based on the number of performance criteria written that are associated with a scoring strategies. For example, if four scoring levels are used, the total criterion value (second column) must equal 25 and the ideal performance score must be four ($4 \times 25 = 100$). If a total of four scoring strategies were being used, the scores would range from one to four. If only three were needed, the scores would range from two to four. However, if five scoring strategies are being used, the total criterion value must be adjusted to equal 20 and the ideal performance, five ($5 \times 20 = 100$). The lower performance scores would then be one through five.

To summarize, when grading a student's assignment, the weight of the criterion value (row) is multiplied by the scoring strategy for the column (top of column) that best describes the student's performance. For example, if a student scored at the advanced beginner level (three points) for the first criterion, which carries a weight of six points, that student's total score would be 18 points (3×6) for that criterion.

The purpose in having the ideal performance equal 100% is strictly to arrive at a percentage that simplifies the math when computing the final

EXHIBIT 9.3
Scoring Strategy With Weighted Criteria

Performance Criteria	Criterion Value	Accomplished Novice 2 points	Advanced Beginner 3 points	Competent 4 points	Total points
Criterion 1	6	Performance descriptor Criterion 1	Quality definition Criterion 1	Quality definition Criterion 1	
Criterion 2	7	Performance descriptor Criterion 2			
Criterion 3	5	Performance descriptor Criterion 3			
Criterion 4	4	Performance descriptor Criterion 4			
Criterion 5	3	Performance descriptor Criterion 5			
	25			Earned percentage	
				Potential points for assignment	
				Earned points	

EXHIBIT 9.4
How the Analytic Rubric Works

Performance Criteria	Criterion Value	Accomplished Novice 2 points	Advanced Beginner 3 points	Competent 4 points	Total %
Criterion 1	6	Quality definition Criterion 1	Quality definition Criterion 1 3	Quality definition Criterion 1	18
Criterion 2	7	Quality definition Criterion 2	Quality definition Criterion 2 3	Quality definition Criterion 2	21
Criterion 3	5	Quality definition Criterion 3	Quality definition Criterion 3	Quality definition Criterion 3 4	20
Criterion 4	4	Quality definition Criterion 4	Quality definition Criterion 4	Quality definition Criterion 4 4	16
Criterion 5	3	Quality definition Criterion 5 2	Quality definition Criterion 5	Quality definition Criterion 5	6
	25			Earned percentage	81%
				Potential points for assignment	14
				Earned points	11.3

score for assignments that may not carry the same number of points. For example, SOAP note assignments early in the semester may be allotted five points each, whereas the final note at the end of the semester may be worth 20 points. Weighting of performance criteria gives faculty the flexibility to change not only the area of the assignment that should be worth more points, but also to demonstrate to students where they should be spending most of their time.

This strategy of weighting criteria also supports creation of subcategories for each performance criterion if desired, making the specific elements of performance more explicit for students and grading more objective for faculty. Continuing with our example of a rubric for a SOAP note in an advanced health assessment course, the main categories of performance criteria listed in the far left column might be assigned points as follows: *history* = 12, *exam* = 4, *assessment* = 4, and *overall note* = 5. The 12 points for history may be further subdivided into subcategories such as *attribute of a symptom* (four points), *pertinent ROS* (four points), *pertinent social and family history* (two points), and *medications and allergies* (two points). Although creating subcategories is useful, caution is advised at this juncture, as adding subcategories will increase grading time. Until faculty gain familiarity and comfort using the rubric, keeping the subcategories to a minimum is recommended.

The additional step of weighting the performance criteria and arriving at a percentage is what differentiates this type of analytic rubric from what is commonly seen in the literature. This allows faculty to appraise the relative value of the elements of performance, assign an appropriate point value, and simplify the math to arrive at a grade for the assignment. Weighting the performance descriptors also communicates to students where they should concentrate their efforts. Exhibit 9.4 demonstrates how the analytic rubric works when the performance criteria are weighted.

EXCEL-ERATING THE GRADING PROCESS

Rubrics have won praise for promoting objectivity in assessing students' performance, increasing reliability in grading (Sylvestri & Oescher, 2006), informing students of performance expectations (Newell et al., 2002; Nicholson, Gillis, & Dunning, 2009), but have been criticized for increasing the grading time (Anglin, Anglin, Schumann, & Kaliski, 2008). Mertler (2001) contended that grading with an analytic rubric requires multiple reading of assignments, focusing on one performance criterion with each read. One way to make grading using the rubric more time efficient is to use an Excel spreadsheet, which allows the addition of formulas to automatically compute the score.

The rubric I developed consists of two distinct boxes. The larger is the main rubric where faculty enter a student's score, and the grade is calculated by pre-entered formulas which populate the *Total* column, the final column to the right. The second and smaller box below the main rubric is an abbreviated version of the rubric that is automatically populated with scores as the grading progresses in the main rubric. It is labeled *Student's Feedback*. This abbreviated version can be copied and pasted into an e-mail or inserted at the bottom of a written assignment. As an alternative, a screen shot can be captured and used in a similar fashion.

Overview of the Excel-Based Rubric

The rubric in this format is quite easy to use. However, working on the downloaded version as you read on will help with understanding the functionality. Typing the number in the cell that corresponds to the description that is most consistent with the student's performance (2, 3, or 4 in the example provided) and hitting "enter" on the keyboard will automatically populate the far right Totals column. Be sure to hit "enter" after the last score is typed in or the score will not register, and the total points will not be accurate. If the point value for the assignment being graded has been entered in the space provided in the lower right corner of the grid labeled *Potential points,* not only will the percentage earned be calculated, but also the raw score for the particular assignment.

Overview of Formulas in Excel

For those unfamiliar with how to enter formulas into an Excel spreadsheet, a brief explanation is warranted to be able to replicate the rubric. Be aware that some differences exist in the various versions of Excel so you may need to do additional research if my explanation does not coincide with what you are seeing on your computer screen.

With the rubric visible on your computer screen, click on cell 3K (row 3, column K) in the far right column (also indicated by the white arrow in Figure 9.1). To see the formula that resides in that cell, look at the formula bar to the right of *fx* (indicated by the black arrow in Figure 9.1). The formula you will see is = MAX(E3,G3,I3)*4, which indicates that the highest or maximum score (2, 3, or 4) that is entered in the appropriate column (accomplished novice, advanced beginner, or competent) will be multiplied by the weight for that performance criterion, 4 in this case. The weight can be found in the column to the left labeled *Criterion Value*. The product will be entered in the far right Totals column.

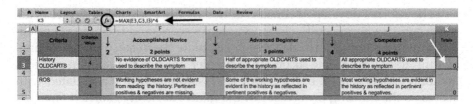

FIGURE 9.1 Formulas Shown in Excel

Try typing in 2, 3, or 4 in the appropriate column for the first criterion, hit "enter" or "return" on your computer, and see the number that appears in the Totals column (far right). For example, if the number 2 had been entered in the corresponding cell under *Accomplished Novice* in the first row for the performance labeled *History OLDCARTS*, the number 8 would appear in the far right column, as this performance criterion carries a weighted score of four. This score will also appear in the same location in the *student's* feedback version of the rubric seen below the main rubric on the Excel sheet.

How to Enter Formulas in Excel

Row Formulas

To enter formulas when creating your own rubric, you first need to be aware of which columns the scores will be added to when grading. In the example provided (Figure 9.2), these are columns E, G, and I. To enter the formula initially, click on the cell where the formula will reside in the Totals column, indicated by the white arrow to the far right in Figure 9.1. Next, click on the dropdown *arrow* to the right of the sigma sign, Σ, in the toolbar

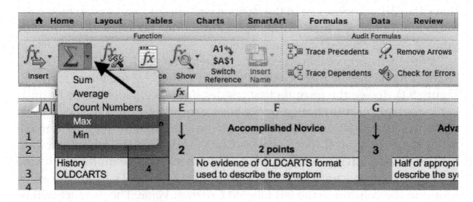

FIGURE 9.2 Adding a Formula in Excel

noted by arrow in Figure 9.2, and choose "MAX." After clicking on MAX, an equal sign will appear in the formula bar to the right of *fx* in front of MAX followed by open and closed parentheses. It will look like this: =MAX().

Depending upon the operating system you use (Windows or OS) and the version of Excel on your computer, what may appear in the *fx* area after =MAX is a formula that includes what may seem like arbitrary cells, with the area encircled with a dotted line in the body of the Excel sheet. That will need to be changed. You can either drag the corners of the dotted line to adjust the cells you want to include in the formula or place the cursor between the parentheses and delete what is there, leaving =MAX() to which you can then add (E3,G3,I3) within the parentheses. Separate each cell indicator with a comma and do not include any spaces. Thus, your final formula for each row (using the appropriate row numbers and column letters) will include no spaces with rows and columns separated with a comma. Each formula will be set up in this format: =MAX(ColumnRow, ColumnRow,ColumnRow)*x, where the asterisk indicates multiplication and the "x" is the weighted value of the criterion value for each row. What this formula does is compute the score for each performance criterion (row).

Adding Row Scores

Since the scoring strategy is based on 100 in this rubric, adding the row scores in the Totals column becomes a percentage. To avoid confusing students, I have labeled this area *Earned percentage*. To add these scores, place your cursor in the cell to the right of the cell labeled *Earned percentage*, which is in the lower right corner of the rubric. Click on the dropdown arrow to the right of the sigma sign (Σ) in the toolbar and choose "SUM" (see Figure 9.2). Delete the formula that appears between the parentheses in the *fx* bar (if one appears) and enter the letter of the Totals column, which is "K" (see Exhibit 9.1), and the row numbers where the scores reside separated by commas. The result shown in Figure 9.3 should look like this =SUM(K3,K5,K7,K9,K11,K13,K15,K17).

Computing the Raw Score

The final formula to be added is one that will multiply the percentage by the point value of the assignment, resulting in the raw score the student earned for the assignment. To add this formula, place your cursor in the cell to the right of the cell labeled *Earned points,* which is in the lower right corner of the rubric. Next, click on the *Formula builder* (black circle in Figure 9.4) and a dropdown screen will appear. Scroll down until you find *PRODUCT* and double click on it. To continue, you will need to close the dropdown screen. Delete what is populated within the parentheses (if anything appears) and add the cell numbers from the Totals column to the right of *Earned*

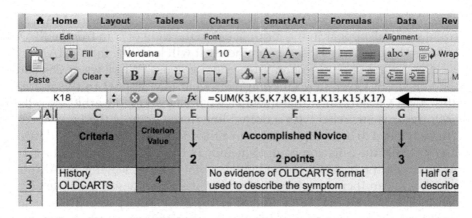

FIGURE 9.3 Sum of Totals in Excel

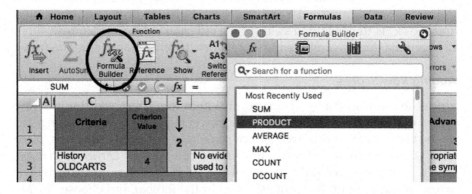

FIGURE 9.4 The Formula Builder in Excel

percentage (K18) and *Potential points* (K19) with a colon separating the two. After the parenthesis, add a forward slash and 100 to arrive at the raw score the student has earned for the assignment. The formula will look like this = PRODUCT(K18:K19)/100 as noted in Figure 9.5. Note that the cell in the Totals column to the right of *Potential points* does not contain a formula. Points can be modified to reflect those allotted to each assignment prior to using the rubric to grade.

Student's Feedback Rubric

The small box that replicates the actual grading in the main rubric can be set up following the same procedure used to add the formulas. The advantage of this set up—a main rubric and the abbreviated rubric—is that you

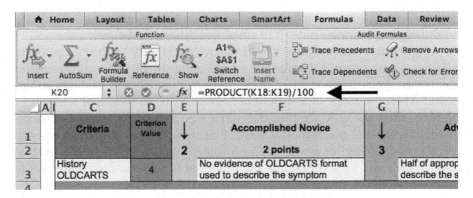

FIGURE 9.5 Computing the Raw Score in Excel

can fill in the main rubric when grading a student's work, which will automatically populate the student's feedback area, copy and paste the student's feedback rubric at the end of the student's assignment, erase the main rubric, and use it again to grade another student. Just be sure to delete the numbers *from the cell in which you added them* and not from the Totals column or you will erase the formulas. The only cell in the Totals column that can be modified without deleting a formula is the *Point value of the assignment*, which can be customized for each assignment.

Creating both a main rubric and student's feedback rubric avoids having to save a copy of the main rubric on your computer for each student. As you will retain a copy of the student's assignment with the smaller version of the student's feedback rubric attached, you will have a record of how the student's work was graded. Should the student challenge his or her grade, you can easily extrapolate how you scored each level of performance from the smaller rubric.

Although no studies have yet to be done on the ability of this format to increase grading efficiency, my experience has been that this method does save time once faculty have worked with it for a while. In addition, students receive the numerical feedback aligned with the performance criteria, which they can then compare with their copy of the rubric to self-assess and determine how their performance was rated.

THE TAKE-AWAY

Rubrics offer an alternative to grading that provides students with specific information on assignment criteria, how points are distributed, and how to earn full points. A well-designed rubric provides a means of increasing faculty's objectivity and interrater reliability when grading. As an addition to the typical scoring strategy in previously published rubrics, the ability to weight each performance criteria provides faculty with the option to change the weight of the criteria for each assignment and indicate to students the relative importance of each criterion. This will help students understand when the focus of assessment has changed, so they will know how to focus their study. Migrating the rubric into an Excel spreadsheet incorporates automatic calculation features that show the points earned on each performance criterion, an overall percentage score, and the final grade on the assignment. This rubric has the potential to save grading time and to improve feedback to students.

REFERENCES

Allen, D., & Tanner, K. (2006). Rubrics: Tools for making learning goals and evaluation criteria explicit for both teachers and learners. *CBE—Life Sciences Education, 5*, 197–203.

Anglin, L., Anglin, K., Schumann, P. L., & Kaliski, J. A. (2008). Improving the efficiency and effectiveness of grading through the use of computer-assisted grading rubrics. *Decision Sciences Journal of Innovative Education, 6*(1), 51–73.

Benner, P. (1984/2001). *From novice to expert: Excellence and power in clinical nursing practice.* Upper Saddle River, NJ: Prentice Hall Health. [Commemorative edition. Original work published 1984]

Bradshaw, J. J., & Lowenstein, A. J. (2011). *Innovative teaching strategies in nursing and related health professions* (2nd ed.). Sudbury, MA: Jones & Bartlett.

Bresciani, M., Zelna, C. I., & Anderson, J. A. (2004). Criteria and rubrics. In M. J. Bresciani, C. L. Zelna, & J. A. Anderson (Eds.), *Assessing student learning and development: A handbook for practitioners* (pp. 29–37). Washington, DC: National Association of Student Personnel Administrators.

Dawson, P. (2015). Assessment rubrics: Towards clearer and more replicable design, research and practice. *Assessment & Evaluation in Higher Education, 42*(3), 347–360. Retrieved from doi:10.1080/02602938.2015.1111294

Gikandi, J. W., Morrowa, D., & Davis, N. E. (2011). Online formative assessment in higher education: A review of the literature. *Computers & Education, 57*, 2333–2351.

Isaacson, J. J., & Stacy, A. S. (2009). Rubrics for clinical evaluation: Objectifying the subjective experience. *Nurse Education in Practice, 9*, 134–140.

Jonsson, A. (2013). Facilitating productive use of feedback in higher education. *Active Learning in Higher Education, 14*(1), 63–76.

Kennedy, K. J., Chan, J. K. S., Fok, P. K., & Yu, W. M. (2008). Forms of assessment and their potential for enhancing learning: Conceptual and cultural issues. *Educational Research for Policy and Practice, 7*(3), 197–207.

Lunney, M., & Sammarco, A. (2009). Scoring rubric for grading students' participation in online discussions. *Computers, Informatics, Nursing, 27*(1), 26–31.

Mertler, C. A. (2001). Designing scoring rubrics for your classroom. *Practical Assessment, Research & Evaluation, 7*(3), 1–8. Retrieved from http://pareonline .net/getvn.asp?v=7&n=25

Milligan, F. (1996). The use of criteria-based grading profiles in formative and summative assessment. *Nurse Education Today, 16,* 413–418.

Moskal, B. M. (2000). Scoring rubrics: What, when and how. *Practical Assessment, Research & Evaluation, 7*(3), 1–5. Retrieved from http://pareonline.net/getvn .asp?v=7&n=3

Moskal, B. M. (2003). Recommendations for developing classroom performance assessments and scoring rubrics. *Practical Assessment, Research & Evaluation, 7*(3), 1–5. Retrieved from http://PAREonline.net/getvn.asp?v=8&n=14

Newell, J. A., Dahm, K. D., & Newell, H. L. (2002). Rubric development and inter-rater reliability issues in assessing learning outcomes. *Chemical Engineering Education, 36*(3), 212–215.

Nicholson, P., Gillis, S., & Dunning, T. (2009). The use of scoring rubrics to determine clinical performance in the operating suite. *Nurse Education Today, 29,* 73–82.

Popham, W. J. (1997). What's wrong—and what's right—with rubrics. *Educational Leadership, 55*(2), 72–75.

Reddy, Y. M., & Andrade, H. (2010). A review of rubric use in higher education. *Assessment & Evaluation in Higher Education, 35*(4), 435–448.

Sadler, D. R. (2010). Fidelity as a precondition for integrity in grading academic achievement. *Assessment & Evaluation in Higher Education, 35*(6), 727–743.

Scanlan, J. M., & Care, W. D. (2004, October). Grade inflation: Should we be concerned? *Journal of Nursing Education, 43*(10), 475–478.

Sylvestri, L., & Oescher, J. (2006). Using rubrics to increase the reliability of assessment in health classes. *International Electronic Journal of Health Education, 9,* 25–30.

Tierny, R., & Simon, M. (2004). What's still wrong with rubrics: Focusing on the consistency of performance criteria across scale levels. *Practical Assessment, Research & Evaluation, 9*(1), 1–7. Retrieved from http://pareonline.net/getvn.asp? v=9&n=2

Truemper, C. M. (2004, December). Using scoring rubrics to facilitate assessment and evaluation of graduate-level nursing students. *Journal of Nursing Education, 43*(12), 562–564.

Wu, S. V., Heng, M. A., & Wang, W. (2015). Nursing students' experiences with the use of authentic assessment rubric and case approach in the clinical laboratories. *Nurse Education Today, 35,* 549–555.

10

Presence in an Online Course

THE COMMUNITY OF INQUIRY MODEL

The model most often cited when discussion turns to presence in the online environment is the community of inquiry (COI) model of Garrison, Anderson, and Archer (1999; see Figure 10.1). This model identifies three interrelated types of presence—social, cognitive, and teaching—that interact to create an online environment to promote learning. To this model, Shea and Bidjerano (2012) proposed adding a fourth presence, that of learning. In this chapter, we explore the COI model, current research, and best practices that the model suggests. We then turn to the more practical side of teaching online and operationalizing the COI in Chapter 11.

My goal in this chapter is not to strictly reiterate the seminal work of Garrison et al. (1999), but instead to provide a stronger case for two perspectives of the COI, that of students as well as faculty. I feel this is important in view of the work of Shea and Bidjerano (2010), who have underscored what the learner brings to the COI. Their suggestion to add a separate presence, that of *learner presence* as the fourth presence in the model, provided insight into the original conceptualization, and allowed me to reflect on aspects that perhaps I had not fully considered. Although the characteristics of the learner are important in terms of creating and maintaining a COI and should have a more prominent position in the model, adding the fourth presence seems to me to muddy the waters. Instead of doing so, I suggest that both learners and faculty share aspects of social, cognitive, and teaching presence that are interdependent and necessary for inquiry to occur.

SOCIAL PRESENCE

Social presence was initially defined as "the ability of participants in the Community of Inquiry to project their personal characteristics into the

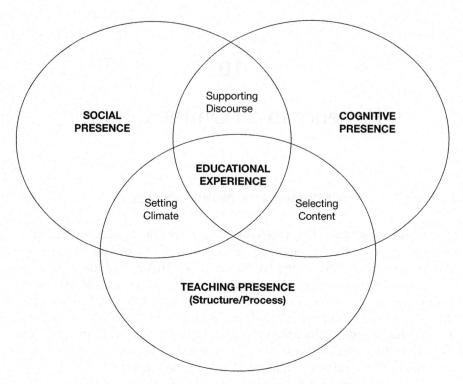

FIGURE 10.1 Community of Inquiry Framework
Source: Garrison (2007). Reprinted by permission of Dr. D. R. Garrison.

community, thereby presenting themselves to the other participants as real 'people'" (Garrison et al., 1999, p. 89). In the early days of online education, a great deal of emphasis was placed on the social aspects of online courses. Some felt that a sense of community, similar to that developed in a classroom setting, would be difficult to replicate online because the subtle nuances that occurred in the classroom, such as eye contact, welcoming smiles, and body language, were absent in the online world (Garrison, Cleveland-Innes, & Fung, 2010; Palloff & Pratt, 2007). However, this has not been shown to be the case after all, as students and faculty found ways to communicate effectively and develop personal connections.

Three indicators of social presence were identified in the COI model according to Garrison et al. (1999, p. 100) and are listed in Box 10.1. The indicators were discussed in this order in the literature, and I believe many felt the order indicated a progression toward social presence—almost a formula of sorts:

Emotional expression + open communication = group cohesion

BOX 10.1
THREE INDICATORS OF SOCIAL PRESENCE
1. Emotional expression (humor and self-disclosure)
2. Open communication (mutual awareness and recognition)
3. Group cohesion

This progression indicated that emotional expression was a precursor to open communication, which was required to develop a sense of group cohesion. However, over time and based on continued research, the relationship of these three indicators shifted, a different temporal relationship emerged, and emotional expression took somewhat of a backseat to open communication and the understood common purpose of learning. Garrison, Cleveland-Innes, et al. (2010) subsequently redefined social presence as "the ability of participants to identify with the community (e.g., course of study), communicate purposefully in a trusting environment, and develop inter-personal relationships by way of projecting their individual personalities" (p. 32) to situate the purpose of the community, that of shared learning, in a prominent place. This corresponds with work of Rogers and Lea (2005), who found that students first identified with the purpose of the course and personal relationships developed as a product of that shared purpose.

The relationship among the three presences—social, cognitive, and teaching—has not been researched as often as each presence separately (Garrison, Anderson, & Archer, 2010), but generally speaking it is the faculty's responsibility to initially set the tone for social presence to develop and support learning (cognitive presence). Strategies to do that follow.

It is easy to forget that in the COI model the term *participant* includes both students and faculty in terms of developing and maintaining social, cognitive, and teaching presence. The three indicators of social presence, expression of emotion, open communication, and group cohesion have different and interdependent implications for students and faculty. The roles students and faculty have in developing social presence differed, however, in timing, focus (monitor vs. monitored), and relationship to cognitive presence.

Most nursing students returning for the RN to bachelor of science in nursing (BSN) degree or entering graduate school instinctively understand why they were there. They are adults who have educational goals in mind and most are self-directed—two assumptions of andragogy (Forrest & Peterson, 2006). Nevertheless, some need guidance in adjusting to the online environment and working collaboratively in groups. The role of faculty in creating social presence has therefore shifted from promoting social relationships to that of creating a safe space where open communication and critical discourse can occur (Garrison & Arbaugh, 2007). For faculty, modeling caring, professional, collegial behavior that creates a *we are in this together* atmosphere underscores the fact that learning is not a one-way street. Modeling also helps to create a safe space in which students are not afraid to post their understandings or make mistakes, allowing them the freedom to learn.

Indicators of Social Presence

Emotional Expression

In the online environment, emotions are expressed by introducing humor and self-disclosure. Faculty must find the balance between sharing too much personal information or humorous anecdotes as if trying to make friends, and seeming too distant, taking the *sage on the stage* stance. Millennial learners relate more effectively to faculty who share who they are, how and why they became educators, and how they balance work and life responsibilities (Roberts, Newman, & Schwartzstein, 2012). In addition, Price (2010) notes that millennials do not do well in an authoritarian power structure, relating better to faculty they perceive as "down-to-earth, informal, relaxed, and flexible" as opposed to those who are "uptight, strict, intimidating, or condescending" (p. 3). They describe their ideal professor as one who is "approachable and easy to talk to'" (p. 4).

Another fairly uncommon occurrence in online discussions, but one that deserves mention, involves students whose posts remain strictly of a social nature that do not contribute to the development of critical discourse. Janssen, Erkens, Kirschner, and Kanselaar (2012) studied the relationship between task and social regulation to overall group performance on a task. They found that task regulation and coordination of group processes and progress positively affected group performance, whereas dialogue of a purely social nature, such as joking, personal disclosure, and indicating agreement or lack of understanding with what the student had posted, had a negative effect. Although this supports what I said earlier, it also underscores the importance of faculty oversight to ensure that social presence in terms of emotional expression tapers off so that cognitive presence can become the prominent feature in online discussions.

Open Communication

Garrison and colleagues (1999) characterized open communication as "reciprocal and respectful exchanges" (p. 100) whose indicators were mutual awareness and recognition. Given that online education is basically a text-based medium, the tone and wording of not only faculty posts and announcements, but also individual e-mails should be approached with care. Phrasing should be upbeat, informal, and begin with a personal salutation (with an individual's name or "For all" in online posts) included. Keep in mind that every piece of written communication is permanent and is an opportunity for faculty to model appropriate online behavior. Although you cannot control how another person perceives something you have written, rereading any written communication will often pick up nuances that could be misunderstood.

Mutual Awareness

Mutual awareness is part of open communication and occurs when responding to students in the discussion, particularly who you choose to respond to and how often you respond. As responding to all students' posts in every discussion is not recommended (see Chapter 11), rotating your replies so that you respond to all students equally throughout the discussions in the course demonstrates awareness of all. If you do not track this, you may find yourself consistently replying to a few students and not to others. A tool to track your responses to students is discussed in Chapter 11.

When a student replies to another student's post, the subtle message is that this student's post has been deemed worthy of reply over the others in the thread. This adds a sense of camaraderie and can be a motivating factor. Students should be instructed to personalize the reply by starting out the post with "Hi, Jane," for example, or adding "Response to Jane" in the subject line, emphasizing the personal connection. This practice, which should be encouraged, is helpful not only to display a sense of mutual awareness, but also to organize the discussion thread so it is clear who is responding to whom. Faculty should do the same when replying to students.

Whenever possible when replying to a student, mention or directly quote something a student has posted that piqued your interest or is particularly relevant to the topic, and expand upon the idea or associate it with content from another student's post. Although this is good practice for faculty, students can overuse this approach and avoid contributing to the discussion, essentially becoming "stuck" in the mutual awareness aspect of social presence. This becomes evident when a student's reply to a classmate includes only direct quotes from his or her post or paraphrases what they had posted. Although this is an excellent means of showing mutual support, without the replier adding additional content or asking a question to advance the conversation, the discussion will stagnate. Students who repeatedly use this approach may be disengaged in the discussion, lack preparation, or do not have an understanding of course content. For that reason, discussion posts, especially early on in the course, must be carefully monitored for ongoing social behavior, as some behaviors are useful, whereas others can impede the discourse from shifting to collaborative critical inquiry.

Recognition

Recognition, the other aspect of open communication, is demonstrated when students acknowledge the value of others' contributions and show agreement with and appreciation for their perspectives. Faculty can demonstrate recognition by starting their posts with "I so appreciate that you mentioned . . ." or "I agree with your comment regarding . . .," which provides encouragement that will impact motivation and persistence. Although this aspect of presence is important to the development of a cohesive community, sustaining it is more important (and perhaps essential) if the content of the discussion relates to the affective domain rather than the cognitive. However, if the goal of the discussion is knowledge construction, continued reliance on this approach when replying to a post can be deleterious to the outcome for the entire group. Without adding a substantive comment, additional related content, or asking a probing question, posts that only reiterate what the other student has said or are strictly complimentary do not move the discussion forward. Do keep in mind that this type of behavior may indicate that the student does not understand the content being discussed, a red flag that his or her zone of proximal development has been encountered. In this instance, scaffolding from faculty may be the best choice of action (see Chapter 11) from a pedagogical perspective.

Posts indicating that the student is stuck in the open communication phase of social presence are easy to miss, but perilous to the outcome of the discussion, as well as the potential learning of the responding student. The concern is that other students will follow suit and take up this rather easy means of getting credit for posts. The best approach for faculty is to privately e-mail any student who demonstrates continued and *exclusive* use of mutual awareness and/or recognition when replying to a classmate's post to problem solve, clear up any misconceptions regarding the quality of postings, point out exemplars of "good" posts within the discussion, and reiterate that the goal of knowledge construction requires substantive posts— or whatever wording is included in your grading rubric that addresses the quality of student's responses. From my perspective, the term *substantive* refers to the depth of the post and demonstrates higher cognitive functioning of application, analysis, synthesis, or evaluation of course content.

Students who persist in demonstrating this type of social behavior will require continued and close monitoring, and perhaps continued private feedback, until they move on to more of a collaborative type of knowledge construction. My experience in teaching graduate students indicated that this behavior is not common, but I did not want to overlook it. The discussion-tracking tool is useful in helping me remember which student is exhibiting continued social presence so I can intervene as necessary.

Group Cohesion

Faculty's role in promoting group cohesion relies, in part, on that of monitoring the quality of students' posts and on the art of facilitation that is discussed in detailed in Chapter 11. Frequent monitoring allows you to guide students so that a discussion is what occurs rather than a series of unrelated narratives. Connecting contents of posts noting either similarities or contrasting features and mentioning student's names and perspectives will help to promote the idea that this is a collaborative effort. Also, bringing in your own perspective and examples from your experience may help students connect and function as a group.

Group cohesiveness is essential if a collaborative group project is the deliverable from the discussion, and necessary if coconstruction of knowledge is the goal. However, achieving these ends is also a function of faculty presence in the course (teaching presence), facilitative abilities, and being aware of and understanding the cognitive level required to complete the activity (i.e., knowledge, comprehension, application, analysis, synthesis, or evaluation). I have witnessed instances in which discussions did not involve any integration because the discussion question was written at the knowledge or comprehension level of Bloom's taxonomy. Because of this, students simply paraphrased information from their textbooks, resulting in every post containing the same content—a series of monologues as noted by Garrison et al. (1999). When this occurs, there is simply nothing to discuss, and students struggle to find ways to contribute to and maintain a discussion. Discussion questions aimed at the lower cognitive levels of Bloom (knowledge and comprehension) actually increased cognitive load (Chapter 1).

Course Design to Promote Social Presence

Features of course design that can promote development of social presence early on include an online forum (discussion group link) dedicated to introductions within the assigned small discussion groups if the class is large, or for the entire class if the number of students is more manageable. A class of 25 to 30 students can all introduce themselves in one link. If separate discussion forums are set up for this purpose, allowing members of other groups to peek in and join the introductions if they so desire is a good plan. The forum for introductions should be opened when the class starts, as students are often eager to get started and may feel a bit intimidated by posting online if the course occurs early in their academic program. Faculty should be active in this area and welcome students one by one or by grouping names in one post. It is essential to respond to the student by name, starting your post with "Hello, Mary," "Hi, Mary," or just "Mary," although the latter seems a bit harsh. In large-enrollment classes where this approach is not feasible, periodically posting how much you are enjoying learning about each student and thanking them for introducing themselves will transmit the message that you are reading the introductions. Remember to use emoticons effectively to transmit feelings if the words alone do not capture them.

Although this forum provides a place for students and faculty to get acquainted, it also gives students a chance to experiment with posting in a discussion where no evaluation of their post will occur. If your course occurs early on in the academic program, structuring the introductions by providing questions for students to respond to will be welcomed. In my experience, I have not witnessed much interaction in the introductory postings, but students do share information about their personal and professional lives, so that other students have a sense of who their classmates are in terms of nursing specialty, experience, and personal interests.

Keep in mind that introductions are not an element of academic achievement (Chapter 9) so no points should be allotted to this activity. This is one course activity that is optional. However, in my experience, most, if not all, students do take the time to post an introduction.

Although the defining factors of the social aspect of online education have changed somewhat over the years, its relationship to cognitive presence remains foundational. Learners who cannot collaborate or cooperate and do not share a common goal will have difficulty developing a sense of community, where inquiry is central (Garrison, 2007).

COGNITIVE PRESENCE

Cognitive presence has been defined in a number of ways over the years, but the most meaningful definition, in my view, was offered by Garrison (2007) as "the exploration, construction, resolution and confirmation of understanding through collaboration and reflection in a community of inquiry" (p. 65). This is based on Dewey's practical inquiry model as conceptualized for teaching online by Garrison and colleagues (1999). The four steps in the inquiry process model are listed in Box 10.2.

In the first step of Dewey's inquiry model as conceptualized by Garrison and colleagues (1999), a triggering event starts the discussion and is often posed in the form of a question to be answered or a problem to be solved.

BOX 10.2
THE FOUR STEPS IN THE INQUIRY PROCESS MODEL
1. Triggering event
2. Exploration
3. Integration
4. Resolution or "application of an idea" or "hypothesis" (Garrison et al., 1999, p. 99) recognizing that not all discussion topics lend themselves to resolution

---

Whatever the format, dissonance, or a sense of imbalance, occurs that must be resolved (Garrison et al., 1999). Although faculty typically start the discussion with a triggering event, as the discussion evolves students may post questions to faculty or in reply to classmates that stimulate a new and appropriate direction of inquiry. Indicators of this phase are posts that reflect "puzzlement" or "recognition of the problem" (Akyol & Garrison, 2011, p. 240).

The exploration phase is signaled by "divergence, information exchange, suggestions, and brainstorming" (Akyol & Garrison, 2011, p. 240). During this phase students search the literature and ideally analyze, synthesize, and evaluate what they have found, reflecting on it in order to formulate a post and reply to classmates to compare and contrast perspectives.

In the integration phase, students reflect on their ideas and the ideas of others to arrive at a perspective that makes sense to them. Indicators of this phase are "convergence, synthesis, and solutions" (Akyol & Garrison, 2011, p. 240). As students post their understanding, the dialogue continues and additional insights may be gained. Depending upon the nature of the discussion topic, question, or problem, faculty may decide to end the discussion at the end of this phase with each student then submitting an assignment that provides his or her perspective toward resolution. This approach is often taken in discussions of clinical cases, where faculty prefer that each student develop his or her own plan of care as a summative assessment.

The resolution phase (or application of an idea) and final phase of the practical inquiry process is one in which "apply, test, and defend" (Akyol & Garrison, 2011, p. 240) are indicators. How the process of resolution occurs is once again dependent upon the nature of the triggering event. Many cases in nursing are ill structured and messy (terms discussed in Chapter 2) and no resolution or final answer is sought. Learning occurs during the *process* of discourse as divergent explanations are discussed and students defend their ideas. The result is often an off-line reflection on the conversation with students arriving at their own conclusions. In this type of situation and after the discussion ends, it is often helpful for faculty to summarize the points made, compare and contrast their validity, and offer an opinion as to what he or she would have done to address the situation or resolve the problem presented.

Although this process certainly appears to be linear, I propose that it is circuitous or resembles a spiral, as students respond to the original discussion question posted by faculty and work through the steps, but then raise questions of their own during discourse, which then go through the same step-wise inquiry process. Early studies demonstrated that discussions did not reach the integration and resolution phase, which was thought to be due to the type of question posed (in terms of levels of Bloom) and the level and frequency of teaching presence (Garrison, Anderson, & Archer, 2001).

Faculty Roles

The faculty role in cognitive presence is difficult to separate from that of teaching presence, so perhaps reviewing the student-focused definition of cognitive presence again will be helpful. Recall that Garrison's (2007) definition involved "the exploration, construction, resolution and confirmation of understanding through collaboration and reflection in a community of inquiry" (p. 65). Here the faculty role relates to cognition as well, and is one of monitoring the discussion, reflecting on students' posts, and devising responses that will validate, encourage, and move the discussion forward. This occurs via facilitative strategies and perhaps direct instruction that falls under teaching presence, which is discussed in the next main section (Teaching Presence).

The role faculty plays in creating the *triggering event*—the discussion questions or cases—cannot be overemphasized, for it is the type and level of questions that will engender a certain level of response and will determine the type and depth of learning that will occur. Developing engaging discussion questions or cases that not only help to assess the objectives, but also provide context and content that lead to coconstruction of knowledge become the main source for learning and assessment. Even in discussions in which students will lead, faculty should be involved in developing the discussion question or problem—the triggering event—so that it contributes to assessing the course objectives. Chapter 7 is devoted to the process of writing these high-level discussion questions and Chapter 6 to writing cases.

During the exploration phase, faculty's role is to simply lurk in the background of the discussion, observing the direction the discussion is taking, at least until all students in each small discussion group have posted initially. If faculty intervene too early, they risk hijacking the discussion with students developing expectations that faculty now have the lead in providing answers and direction. This is a time when faculty should sit on their hands, so to speak, and simply observe or what is referred to as *lurk* in the discussion.

During the integration and resolution phases, teaching presence takes over. At this juncture, the role of faculty is to monitor the quality of the discussion and be sure students progress through the three subsequent stages of the critical inquiry process, remain on topic, and stay on track to achieve the desired learning outcomes. Skillfully facilitating the discussion as it progresses becomes a balance of lurking, posing probing questions, asking for clarification, teaching directly when needed, and providing encouragement. Knowing which strategy to use is discussed in Chapter 11.

Student Roles

As mentioned earlier, the definition of *cognitive presence* describes what the learner will do, which relies somewhat upon faculty's ability to facilitate the process. The roles students play in cognitive presence can be seen as aligned with the ideas of Shea and Bidjerano (2010), who have conceptualized a fourth element of the COI, that of learning presence.

In order for students to explore, construct, resolve, and confirm understanding, they must have some level of skill to self-regulate, which requires planning, monitoring, and reflection, as well as metacognitive and motivational strategies. Students in any given online course will, of course, vary in these skills, but the nursing students most likely taking online courses—RNs seeking a bachelor degree in nursing or enrolling in a graduate program—have already demonstrated these skills to some degree. Thus, an interdependent role of students and faculty plays out in online discussions.

TEACHING PRESENCE

Teaching presence has been defined as "the design, facilitation, and direction of cognitive and social processes for the purpose of realizing personally meaningful and educationally worthwhile learning outcomes" (Garrison et al., 2007, p. 163). Teaching presence is comprised of the three categories listed in Box 10.3. Although this definition is teaching-focused, it is not necessarily teacher-focused. Elements of facilitating discourse and direct instruction are not restricted to faculty assigned to teach the course. Students can, and often do, take on these roles (Garrison et al., 1999).

> **BOX 10.3**
> **CATEGORIES OF TEACHING PRESENCE**
>
> 1. Instructional design and management
> 2. Facilitating discourse
> 3. Direct instruction

Faculty Roles

Instructional Design and Management

Research has shown that providing clear and consistent course structure is the most reliable predictor of successful online courses (Garrison & Arbaugh, 2007). *Instructional design and management* encompasses planning activities before the course begins and throughout the duration of the course. Precourse design includes (a) structuring the course by identifying outcomes (course objectives), assessments, and teaching strategies (Backward Design, Chapter 3); (b) organizing the online course management system (Chapter 12) so it is intuitive, aligns with the course syllabus, and navigation does not interfere with learning; and (c) assuming leadership in organizing faculty if the course is cotaught. From an instructional design perspective, management during the course involves continual monitoring and rapid response to unanticipated technical problems. After the course is completed, grades must be posted, and both students' end-of-course survey results and faculty's reflection on the course itself must be considered in terms of identifying potential areas for revision before the course is taught again.

Facilitating Discourse

Facilitating discourse is the process of guiding students through the four phases of the critical inquiry process (Garrison et al., 1999), shaping the discussion without being at the center of it, and ensuring that outcomes are met through indirect and unobtrusive assistance. In this definition, the words indirect and unobtrusive are key. *Indirect* differentiates facilitation (taking the role of guide) from that of direct instruction in which information or the answer is given. Guidance can be provided in the form of a probing question, linking content together, or connecting the ideas in two or more student's posts, all done with the intention of allowing students to *uncover* the right path or information (see Backward Design, Chapter 3). The term unobtrusive speaks for itself and what it implies has been mentioned previously. Faculty's role in discussions must remain fairly transparent.

I think the term *catalyst* applies here in that faculty's role should be that of moving the discourse forward without taking control or really being noticed. Facilitation, I believe, is an art that can be learned. Specific facilitation strategies are discussed in Chapter 11.

Direct Instruction

Direct instruction occurs when faculty "provide intellectual and scholarly leadership and share their subject matter knowledge with students" (Anderson, Rourke, & Garrison, 2001, para. 25). This can be accomplished by using techniques from the cognitive apprenticeship model of Collins, Brown, and Holum (1991) such as modeling, scaffolding, fading, and coaching. Chapter 2 discusses the model in greater detail.

Direct instruction can also be delivered by lecture in addition to and outside of the discussion. Suffice to say that lengthy, content-laden lecturing does not translate well to the online environment. Mini lectures have a place when teaching online to cover important or complex topics, but should be short and to the point. Carefully crafted discussion questions in which students can *uncover* the knowledge and understandings through collaborative discussions, independent research, and reflection, mindfully facilitated by faculty will allow most content to come to light, especially if faculty are guided by the cognitive case map for the discussion (see Chapter 6).

According to Garrison and Arbaugh (2007), the timing of feedback and whether facilitation or direction instruction is employed is of utmost importance to meeting students' needs. Knowing when to facilitate and when to teach will come with online teaching experience. Facilitation, in my opinion, encourages construction and coconstruction of knowledge more effectively than direction instruction *unless* the student has entered his or her zone of proximal development, and it is obvious that asking the student a probing question will not help. When sensing students' frustration, it is essential that the emotion is recognized and faculty voice their understanding and willingness to help in order to calm them and provide customized direction to help them move forward and learn.

The frequency of facilitation or direct instruction in an online discussion is a rather hot topic in educational circles. By frequently and consistently reviewing students' posts and posting at fairly regular intervals, faculty will let their presence be known without taking over the discussion. This topic is discussed in greater detail in Chapter 11.

Student Roles

Although students typically are not given a role in course design, asked to coteach unless assigned to facilitate a discussion, or expected to direct cognitive and social processes, these activities sometimes naturally occur. Nursing is such a heterogeneous profession that I am continually amazed at the variety of nursing roles and the vast years of experience of some of my students. Reading their introductions at the onset of the course is often enlightening—and sometimes intimidating. Nursing is frequently a second career choice; thus, students taking an online graduate course may already hold an advanced degree in another field. Also, some students have decades of nursing experience in a variety of roles, whereas others have just graduated with a BSN. Both novices and experts could and most likely will be in the same course and in the same discussion group. I mention this because it is relevant, as students can inadvertently take on elements of teaching presence when it is not a part of your course plan, such as suddenly taking over and leading a discussion.

Students will often pose a probing question in the discussion in response to something another student had posted. Although this will often move the discussion forward or expand it, sometimes it becomes a tangent—a road you do not want students to go down—as it is not a desired outcome of the discussion. Also, students may occasionally provide answers to questions posed by faculty or another student that instead of continuing the dialogue stops it in its tracks. This may be a situation in which direct instruction was used when facilitation would have been a better approach. Responding to these attempts to promote knowledge and encourage discussion will require a fair amount of finesse on your part to remedy the situation without offending or embarrassing the student involved. Sometimes simply redirecting the discussion by asking students to postpone discussion on a topic or mentioning that you would rather have them focus their attention on another aspect is sufficient. And, sometimes a private e-mail to the well-intended, yet offending, student is required.

INTERSECTION OF THE PRESENCES

Although the three types of presence—social, teaching, and cognitive—can be discussed as separate entities from a theoretical perspective, they are intertwined in practice. Clearly, some level of social presence in terms of comfort with one another must be established in order for students to feel safe putting their thoughts out in the open in a discussion for critique. Faculty can help to make the learning space feel safe through open and honest communication, providing clear expectations of students, and becoming a real person in the students' eyes by sharing aspects of his or her life. Garrison and Arbaugh (2007) took the interaction of the presences a bit farther, describing the relationship among all three: "Social presence lays the groundwork for higher level discourse; and the structure, organization, and leadership associated with teaching presence creates the environment where cognitive presence can be developed" (p. 163).

THE TAKE-AWAY

The COI model provides the framework for online course design as well as guidance for faculty to help students reach the desired learning goals. Inherent in the model is the idea that both students and faculty can take on the three types of presence, creating somewhat of a dance of teaching and learning.

REFERENCES

Akyol, Z., & Garrison, D. R. (2011). Understanding cognitive presence in an online and blended community of inquiry: Assessing outcomes and processes for deep approaches to learning. *British Journal of Educational Technology, 42*(2), 233–250.

Anderson, T., Rourke, L., & Garrison, D. R. (2001). Assessing teaching presence in a computer conferencing context. *Journal of Asynchronous Learning Networks, 5*(2), 1–17. Retrieved from http://auspace.athabascau.ca/bitstream/2149/725/1/assessing_teaching_presence.pdf

Collins, A., Brown, J. S., & Holum, A. (1991). Cognitive apprenticeship: Making thinking visible. *American Educator, 15*(3), 6–11.

Forrest, S. P., III, & Peterson, T. O. (2006). It's called andragogy. *Academy of Management Learning and Education, 5*(1), 113–122.

Garrison, D. R. (2007). Online community of inquiry review: Social, cognitive, and teaching presence issues. *Journal of Asynchronous Learning Networks, 11*(1), 61–72.

Garrison, D. R., Anderson, T., & Archer, W. (1999). Critical inquiry in a text-based environment: Computer conferencing in higher education. *Internet and Higher Education, 2*(2–3), 87–105.

Garrison, D. R., Anderson, T., & Archer, W. (2001). Critical thinking and computer conferencing: A model and tool to assess cognitive presence. *American Journal of Distance Education, 15*(1), 7–23.

Garrison, D. R., Anderson, T., & Archer, W. (2010). The first decade of the community of inquiry framework: A retrospective. *Internet and Higher Education, 13*, 5–9.

Garrison, D. R., & Arbaugh, J. B. (2007). Researching the community of inquiry framework: Review, issues, and future directions. *Internet and Higher Education, 10*, 137–172.

Garrison, D. R., Cleveland-Innes, M., & Fung, T. S. (2010). Exploring causal relationships among teaching, cognitive and social presence: Student perceptions of the community of inquiry framework. *Internet and Higher Education, 13*, 31–36.

Janssen, J., Erkens, G., Kirschner, P. A., & Kanselaar, G. (2012). Task-related and social regulation during online collaborative learning. *Metacognition and Learning, 7*(1), 25–43.

Palloff, R. M., & Pratt, K. (2007). Building online learning: Effective strategies for the online classroom. San Francisco, CA: Jossey-Bass.

Price, C. (2010). Why don't my students think I'm groovy?: The new "R"s for engaging millennial learners. *Essays From Excellence in Teaching, 9*, 29–34.

Roberts, D. H., Newman, L. R., & Schwartzstein, R. M. (2012). Twelve tips for facilitating Millennials' learning. *Medical Teacher, 34*, 274–278.

Rogers, P., & Lea, M. (2005). Social presence in distributed group environments: The role of social identity. *Behavior & Information Technology, 24*(2), 151–158.

Shea, P., & Bidjerano, T. (2010). Learning presence: Towards a theory of self-efficacy, self-regulation, and the development of communities of inquiry in online and blended learning environments. *Computers & Education, 55*, 1721–1731.

11

Facilitation Strategies and Pearls

From the students' perspective within the community of inquiry (COI) model (Garrison & Arbaugh, 2007), effective teaching presence influences overall satisfaction, perceived learning, and sense of community. In the online environment within discussion boards, where the learning takes place, direct teaching and facilitation are the key faculty strategies that serve to move the discussion through the phases of critical inquiry and to support coconstruction of knowledge. Describing the types of facilitation, understanding the roles of the educator when teaching online, and developing effective facilitation strategies that can be implemented in a transparent manner are an art and the focus of this chapter.

MEANING OF *FACILITATION*

Facilitation allows faculty to drive and shape the discussion without being at the center of it, moving the students toward understanding. Garrison and Arbaugh (2007) explained the requirements:

> Facilitating discourse requires the instructor to review and comment upon student responses, raise questions and make observations to move discussions in a desired direction, keep discussion moving efficiently, draw out inactive students, and limit the activities of dominating posters when they become detrimental to the learning of the group. (p. 164)

Formative feedback occurs in the process of facilitation. Recall that formative feedback is feedback *for* learning, whose goal is to move students toward deeper learning and to meet desired outcomes. While reviewing students' posts and employing facilitative strategies, faculty are also evaluating students' understanding of the content based on the discussion questions (DQs) map (see Chapter 7), which includes specific outcomes of each discussion. In fact, any strategy faculty uses to move the discussion forward or deeper will be with predetermined outcomes in mind.

WHAT FACILITATION IS NOT

Garrison, Anderson, and Archer (1999) differentiated between facilitation and direct instruction, an important distinction. In other words, facilitation does not involve offering additional information in response to the content of a post or directly answering a question posed by a student. While that approach is sometimes useful and appropriate, it is not considered facilitation. One of the benefits of the text-based nature of online education, and posting in discussions in particular, according to Hmelo-Silver and Barrows (2006) is to "place the students' knowledge in public view and help them see the limits of their understanding" (p. 29), allowing them to self-correct or others in the discussion group to suggest an alternative explanation.

TYPES OF INTERACTIONS

In the early days of distance education, Moore (1989) clarified the meaning of *interaction* by defining three types of communication patterns: *learner–content, learner–instructor,* and *learner–learner.* This was undertaken because at the time, distance education was not well defined and consisted of correspondence courses, television-based courses, e-mail, and synchronous chats in which minimal interaction took place with the instructor and limited interaction between and among learners occurred.

The learner–content interaction is at the foundation of learning and adult education, which Moore (1989) described as the "process of intellectually interacting with content that results in changes in the learner's understanding, the learner's perspective, or the cognitive structures of the learner's mind" (p. 2), possibly a provocative statement at the time, but one that cognitive science now fully supports (Brown, Roediger, & McDaniel, 2014). This type of interaction includes reading and learning from various media in independent study, where both cognitive and metacognitive strategies are employed.

As in the classroom, learner–instructor interaction is an essential component of learning. Moore (1989) described the role of teachers, which is "to stimulate or at least maintain the student's interest in what is to be taught, to motivate the student to learn, to enhance and maintain the learner's interest, including self-direction and self-motivation" (p. 2). Teachers also had the responsibility to "organize students' *application* [emphasis added] of what is to be learned" (p. 2), underscoring not only this important function, but also the desired level of learning. The role of developing assessment strategies and evaluating students' progress toward meeting learning outcomes rounds out the learner–instructor interaction, in which Moore underscores the value of individualized feedback.

Learner–learner interaction is now recognized as the heart and soul of online education, which follows constructivist and social constructivist paradigms. Since Moore's (1989) seminal editorial, research has confirmed the value of coconstruction of knowledge in a COI. And it is through the art of facilitation and instructor–learner interaction that learner-to-learner discourse flourishes, remains purposeful, and ultimately achieves the desired learning outcomes.

LOGISTICS OF FACULTY FACILITATION

Frequency of Facilitation

The question of how to operationalize Moore's three types of interaction effectively and efficiently to maintain balance of students' needs with workload expectations is paramount for educators. Boettcher (2009) suggests using the *rule of thirds*. This rule states that interaction in the discussion board should be:

1. One third learner to content
2. One third learner to learner
3. One third instructor to learner

The number of credit hours for the course will determine how many hours outside of the classroom students are expected to spend reading, researching, and, in terms of online education, composing an initial post and responding to classmates. Posting and being active in the discussion board is equivalent to seat time in the classroom. How much time students spend on preparation is time that you, as faculty, cannot control. How student and faculty workload are computed for a course is discussed in Chapter 3, as it directly affects the amount of content you will have time to teach in a course. Consequently, faculty's concern should be on the ratio of learner–learner and instructor–learner dialogue.

When considering that faculty cannot control time spent in learner–content activities, Boettcher's formula takes on a slightly different meaning. It then appears that time learners spend in discussion and faculty spend responding to students' posts should be equal. However, that is not the intent. For this reason, the recommendation of Burge (2008) is perhaps easier to operationalize. Referred to as the 80/20 approach, the intent is for 80% of the interaction to be learner–learner and 20%, instructor–learner. The rationale behind the limited faculty presence is that posting more often may shift the focus of the discussion to you. You will recognize this is occurring when students respond to your posts more often than their classmates. Another more destructive outcome is that the discussion will come to an abrupt halt as students acquiesce to the expert.

A study by An, Shin, and Lim (2009) provided interesting insight into the effect the frequency of faculty's posts had on students' postings. They divided the study group into three discussion groups in which the frequency of faculty facilitation differed. In Group 1, the instructor responded to each student's initial post and students were to respond to at least two classmates. In Group 2, the instructor responded to each student's initial post, but did not require students to respond to classmates. However, they could respond if they so desired. In Group 3, the instructor did not respond to each student's initial post, but required students to respond to two classmates. The results showed that even though faculty responded to every student's main post, the interaction among students did not increase. Instead, when postings by the instructor were minimal, students' postings of thoughts and opinions increased.

Expectations of Facilitation

This brings up the issue of students' expectations of faculty posting. This topic is a bit of a slippery slope, because faculty are often unhappy with the current recommendations. Rovai (2007) likened posting in an online discussion from the student's perspective to "writing a message, placing it in a bottle, and dropping the bottle in the ocean" (p. 82). Unless faculty comment on a post, students may think it has not been read. However, responding to every post will not promote interaction among students, which is essential for coconstruction of knowledge.

Daily posting by faculty seems to be the recommendation from online teaching experts. Although Boettcher and Conrad (2010) recommended logging into the discussion 4 days each week to review student posts, they note that a daily presence in terms of replying to posts, offering encouragement, and/or posting an announcement is associated with higher student satisfaction. Rovai (2007) concurred with daily review in order to keep up with students' posts, avoiding infrequent, time-consuming marathon sessions to catch up. He also recommended posting at least one message per day in each group's discussion board to communicate to students that their contributions were being recognized. Postings whose intended purpose is to indicate presence need not provide formative feedback and can be as simple as expression of appreciation, agreement, support, and/or encouragement. However, keep in mind that these postings do not take the place of facilitating the discussion.

I must agree that daily review is often the best approach. If there are 25 students in the class, for example, and each is required to post initially in response to the DQ and subsequently reply to two classmates, faculty will have at least 75 posts to read in every discussion over a 10-day to 2-week period. And, students often post more frequently, increasing the volume of posts one must wade through. Because of the volume of posts to be read, I find it useful to categorize the types of responses I can make to student posts.

1. *Supportive posts* serve to acknowledge students' posts and encourage others to comment. Wording like "The discussion is moving along nicely—keep up the good work"; or "Interesting thoughts, Mary, Ted, and Jane. I look forward to hearing what Mike has to say."
2. *Inquiry posts* are posts that ask for clarification, additional information, or point out differing perspectives, asking two or more students to comment. This approach should not take the discussion deeper or in a different direction. Stavredes (2011) referred to this as *weaving*.
3. *Outcome-oriented posts* ask probing or thought-provoking questions to stimulate deeper discussion with the goal for students of meeting the learning outcomes as outlined in the cognitive case map discussed in Chapter 6.

The reason I make this distinction is because all *daily* posts by faculty need not and should not be lengthy. Given the multiple demands placed on faculty's time, it may not be possible to create daily outcome-oriented posts, which are often time consuming to write as they require reading a post, assessing the contents, reflecting on the contents' relationship to learning goals, and composing a reply. However, intermingling supportive, inquiry, and outcome-oriented posts will send the message to students that your presence in their discussions is a daily event. Remember that daily presence communicates to students that you are reading their posts and results in higher student satisfaction with the course (Rovai, 2007), which translates to students being happier with you when the end-of-course surveys come around. This recommendation should be taken to heart. Other means of demonstrating daily course presence are possible, such as posting an announcement or a reply to a student's question in the Cybercafé, which is discussed in Chapter 12.

Because of the volume of posts, checking the discussions daily is beneficial in another way and that is to avoid marathon post-reading sessions. I personally find it discouraging to go into the discussion boards and see that I have 30 unread posts, for example. What typically occurs is that many students require most of the first week allotted for a discussion to complete the readings, assimilate the information, and compose an initial post. Thus, the posts straggle in with most of their initial posts appearing toward the end of that first week. If you start the discussion on a Monday with the initial post due by Friday, you may find yourself reading posts all weekend. And, if you have not replied all week, the students most likely have been wondering where you are. I find that pacing myself by spending an hour or two each day in the discussions, posting a combination of the supportive, inquiry, and outcome-oriented posts keeps me engaged and avoids burnout. Plus, my weekends are not spent reading posts. The discussion-tracking tool helps me keep track of where and what type of posting I have done and is discussed in the section that appears later in this chapter, under Tracking Posts.

Timing of Facilitation

The timing of faculty's posts during the discussion is important. The approach I take when facilitating student discussions and the advice I give to faculty is to sit on your hands early on, avoiding the strong urge to correct misconceptions, or ask probing questions to encourage deeper engagement with the content. I take that approach because students require time the first week of each discussion to read and prepare their initial post, which must be completed by the end of the first week, typically. Until all students in a small group post for the first time, I recommend restricting your type of daily faculty posts to those that are supportive or inquiry-based only. You may also want to mention that additional comments from you will be forthcoming after all students have posted initially.

Having all group members' initial thoughts on the table before faculty step in to ask questions to stimulate deeper discussion will ensure that students who have yet to post will not feel as though they were arriving late to the discussion. I try to wait until students begin replying to each other before stepping in. That is why my advice of sitting on one's hands is necessary, as the temptation to jump in is strong—and faculty often feel guilty not doing so. However, we want students to take the lead and drive knowledge coconstruction unless, of course, their ideas need clarification or additional information to fully understand their perspective. If a student's post contains incorrect information or assumptions, other students within the group will often provide needed clarification or correction. Faculty should allow time for that to occur. Early on in a discussion is also the time when it is obvious by the contents of a student's initial post that he or she has entered the zone of proximal development (ZPD), so lurking in the discussion at this juncture is important. Strategies to help you recognize the ZPD are discussed later in this chapter.

Tracking Posts

Because of the volume of posts that must be read, tracking the timing of the initial post, the timing and number of replies to classmates, and the quality of each post is essential and, if consistently done, is an efficient practice. To do so, I developed a discussion-tracking tool and a system of documentation. This tool can be found in the Appendix (Template 11.1). The students' names are added in the far left column, and two columns are added for each discussion—one for the initial post and one for the reply to classmates' posts. I print this form and use it as a worksheet throughout the course, adding symbols in pencil. It can also be copied into an Excel spreadsheet if you prefer that software. I use the following symbols to indicate performance.

- *Initial post*—When a student's initial post meets criteria to earn all points, I will add a "5" or the highest possible number of points that can be earned to indicate that I do not need to revisit that post for quality. I use lower numbers (0–4) to indicate that additional grading will be necessary. The lower the initial number, the more attention the student's work will receive. As I will typically reply to a student who has not met the quality expectations with an inquiry or outcome-oriented post to give him or her another opportunity to expand or clarify his or her original thinking, I will reread all posts by that student at the end of the discussion. A checkmark next to the number indicates I have replied to that student. Hash marks (one or more) through the checkmark indicate additional times I have responded.
- *Replies to classmates*—In the replies column, I use a series of checkmarks and a +/– system. If a student's reply to a classmate meets the expectations set forth in the rubric, I will place a checkmark in the replies column. Two checkmarks mean that the student has met the expectations of replying to two classmates and the quality of those replies is also on point. If a reply has not met expectations, instead of a checkmark, I will add +/– to indicate that. If I reply to the student who has not met expectations, instead of a forward slash in between the + and –, I will add a checkmark. That indicator will look like this: +√–
- I do not track supportive posts that I make, but I do track inquiry and outcome-oriented posts by indicating "I" or "O" above the checkmark, +√–, or +/– in the replies column.
- I do track when a student replies to one of my posts by adding a hash mark through the checkmark or forward slash.

Examples of this type of documentation on a discussion-tracking tool are shown in Exhibit 11.1.

EXHIBIT 11.1
Discussion-Tracking Tool

Name of Students	Discussions									
	1		2		3		4		5	
	I	R	I	R	I	R	I	R	I	R
Joe	5	✓✓								
Mary	o 3	+/.								
Jane	5	7.✓								
Tom	5	✓ 7-								
Helen	I 2	7.								
Elena	5	7. ✓								

I, initial post; R, response post.

Note: See the Appendix for a blank version of this template.

You may find a system that works better for you. However, keep in mind that you want to keep track of:

- *Initial posts*—timing and quality according to your rubric
- *Replies to classmates*—number, timing, and quality according to the rubric
- *Replies to you*—to track students' response to your posts. This should not be counted as one of the required replies to classmates, so you may want to make that clear in the rubric and in an announcement prior to the first few discussions.
- *Whom you reply to*—you want to spread out your replies so that all students receive equal attention and feedback throughout the discussions in the course. This reflects mutual awareness and recognition of social presence (Garrison et al., 1999).
- *Type of post*—inquiry or outcome-oriented

ASSESSING WHAT IS GOING ON IN A DISCUSSION

Student Issues

Key to choosing the appropriate facilitation strategy is accurately assessing what is occurring in the discussions. Questions to ask are listed in Box 11.1. These questions and other student issues are discussed in this section.

BOX 11.1
ASSESSING WHAT IS OCCURRING IN THE DISCUSSIONS

Questions to ask:

- Do students' posts reflect an understanding of the content?
- Are students responding to the DQ at the level required?
- Are they demonstrating the use of higher cognitive functions in their responses?
- Is there evidence of their perspective in their posts, or do they include only that of published authors?

DQ, discussion question.

Indicators of the Struggling Student

At the outset of their program, students who may have returned to school after many years or those who are unaccustomed to the quality of work expected at the graduate level may need careful monitoring and additional guidance in the discussions, especially if your course is early on in their academic program. Just the relatively simple act of applying what they have read to the question at hand, composing their thoughts, and actually writing full sentences may be a struggle initially, especially for those who are accustomed to keeping it brief in text messages and Tweets. Indications that a student is struggling may be reflected in a post that is composed of:

- A series of quotes from published authors without application, analysis, synthesis, or evaluation by the student
- A series of paraphrased content that is all appropriately cited, indicating the thoughts belong to others. Although this indicates students are aware of giving credit where credit is due and the correct American Psychological Association (APA) format, it may also indicate that they do not understand what they are reading and are unable to synthesize others' thoughts and arrive at their own perspective.
- What I have come to call the *blah-blah-blah* post—a post that makes little sense—and in which it is clear that the student does not understand the content, has not had or taken the time to do so, or indicates the student has entered the ZPD.
- Scholarly writing suspicious for plagiarism that seems outside of the ability of the student's educational level

All of these issues require faculty intervention, and all but the plagiarism issue can be addressed in the public arena. Plagiarism is a special case, so I address it first.

Plagiarism

If faculty suspect that work a student is calling his or her own, that is, the work does not include citations and belongs to a published author, validating your suspicions is the first step. Some schools have authenticity software, such as Turnitin, that can compare what a student has written with published works. Free plagiarism-checking software is available online, such as Grammarly, but there are many others. Dropping a suspect sentence or two into the software will tell the tale by citing the original source and showing the passage in context. Likewise, the same method can be used in Google or Google Scholar to locate the original source of content that should have been quoted and properly cited.

Most schools and universities have a strict plagiarism policy and process for academic dishonesty, the umbrella term for plagiarism. Your first step, however, is contacting the student via e-mail or phone to share your concerns. Here I must caution you that they are innocent until proven guilty, so a stance of inquiry will garner more information than one of condemnation. My experience has been that what we recognize as plagiarism is often an honest mistake on the student's part, especially early on in their program.

Students often do not understand the subtle difference when lifting another's words verbatim between two types of citations: (a) citing the author's name and year of publication, or (b) using quotations around the author's words with a citation that includes the authors name, year of publication, and a page or paragraph number. So, that is the first question I ask them: "When would you use quotation marks?" When they cannot explain the difference, I explain it to them and point out the specific concern I have with their work. To some degree, going through this process over the phone or via e-mail places faculty at a disadvantage, as facial expressions and eye cues are not available to help you understand what really happened. However, just mentioning to students that you think they plagiarized often brings gasps, rapid-fire explanations, and tears. Some students become indignant and are aghast that you would even think that of them.

If you believe this incident was an honest mistake, the student's future work will require continued scrutiny, which can be tracked using the discussion-tracking tool (see Exhibit 11.1). You may be required by the school's academic dishonesty policy to inform the academic dean or program chair, so be sure you are aware of what is required.

Deep Versus Surface Learning in a Discussion

Keep in mind that the purpose of discussions, the main learning space in online courses, is to support students' deep learning so what they learn can be transferred to life and the workplace. Recall from Chapter 1 that *surface* learning is associated with memorization, whereas *deep* learning involves learning for understanding. However, discriminating surface from deep learning in discussion posts can be difficult. Entwistle and Waterson (1988, as cited in Offir, Lev, & Bezalel, 2008) compiled a list of indicators of surface and deep interaction that will help faculty delimit them.

Surface-level cognitive processing includes:

- Quoting a published author without interpretation
- Borrowing ideas from classmates' posts without commenting or advancing the conversation
- Proposing a solution without supporting data or rationales
- Proposing more than one solution without indicating one that is preferred
- Asking irrelevant questions that are difficult to associate with the issue at hand

Deep cognitive processing, on the other hand, involves:

- Analyzing, synthesizing, and evaluating new information as it applies to the issue
- Synthesizing new information to arrive at a new approach to the problem
- Proposing solutions indicating the pros and cons of each
- Providing examples to validate proposed solutions
- Approaching a problem from a wider perspective

Supporting deep learning strategies can be managed within the discussion itself using various facilitation techniques that are discussed later in this chapter.

Direct Teaching Versus Facilitation—Which Is Needed?

The main issue faculty face in discussion boards when questions arise or students' understanding is in question is recognizing when to facilitate and when direct teaching is required. Faculty who have taught in the classroom and employed lecture as the main teaching method may be particularly sensitive to the need to provide direct answers to questions or to jump in and seize that teachable moment when facilitation that promotes construction of knowledge is a more appropriate response. How do you know which approach is best in any given situation?

When discussions are set up so that students must each post initially in their discussion group and respond to classmates a specified number of times in order to earn all points for the discussion, you want to give students an opportunity to do just that. Remember that you want to encourage student–student and student–content interactions. Students will often respond and ask each other the necessary questions or correct inaccurate information without faculty intervention. However, if they do not do so after a few days, it is then time for faculty to use facilitation techniques that will provide guidance. Even if a student has asked a direct content-related question, it should not be answered directly—at least not at first. Faculty can provide guidance that will allow the student to connect the dots, such as linking the topic with prior knowledge or other content, or asking meta-cognitive questions that an expert might ask when wrestling with the issue. This is discussed in greater detail in the Facilitation Strategies section that follows. However, at the end of my post in response to a student's question I will typically ask if what I have said makes sense and encourage the student to continue the dialogue. In other words, let the student know that this is just the beginning of the conversation and that you encourage it to continue. I also include a note to others in the discussion to chime in if they wish.

Suffice to say that direct instruction should be the last resort. However, keep in mind that the student's puzzlement may indicate that the ZPD has been entered and the student is at a loss to understand. This is where learner-centered, customized facilitation or direct teaching can and should occur (Reigeluth, 1999). If the student does not respond to your questions posted in the discussion, following up with a private e-mail may be in order. The student may be frustrated by your response or having difficulty with the content. An e-mail will open the door for private dialogue. And, the end result may be that you will need to provide the information the student is missing or indicate a resource where the student can read more about it. Sometimes, it is just reading the information more than once or hearing it in another's words or from a different author's perspective that makes the difference.

FACILITATION STRATEGIES

A variety of facilitation strategies can be employed to support students' construction and coconstruction of knowledge such as questioning, challenging, modeling metacognitive strategies, pushing for elaboration, revoicing, scaffolding, and summarizing. Keep in mind that if students are required to respond to classmates, they may adopt facilitation strategies modeled by faculty. It is hoped that exploring each method in detail will provide multiple strategies for your facilitation toolbox.

Methods of Questioning

Requesting Clarification

The facilitative strategy of questioning can take several forms: requesting clarification, Socratic questioning to make students' thinking visible, and metacognitive questioning. Asking for clarification, if needed, is a quick way to let students know you read their posts. An effective way of doing so in reply to a student is to quote directly from their post and ask them to explain or clarify. Including your understanding of what was said will give the student an opportunity to agree or disagree, and perhaps offer an avenue for deeper exploration. This method is an effective means to learn what the student understands and push him or her toward deeper understanding of the content or issue being discussed. Stavredes (2011) suggested that asking for clarification if a student's post is off topic will help him or her realize the error and reconnect with the topic.

Socratic Method

The Socratic method is a means of questioning whose goal is for students to understand what they know, when that knowledge ends, and the thought processes they use to reason. From the faculty perspective, Socratic questioning helps to delimit the student's ZPD by taking him or her to the boundary of understanding, exposing gaps, demonstrating the student's ability to think critically, and unmasking faulty reasoning (Oh, 2005). However, Socrates often left his students wondering about the answers to the staged questions he asked, which for our purposes in an online environment may not be the best strategy. Questions can be posed, but if the student does not respond, faculty will never know how much learning actually occurred. Consequently, the questions must be carefully worded and asked with the purpose of encouraging deeper learning and meeting intended outcomes through reflection and additional research. To be avoided at all costs is using this type of questioning for a "guess what I'm thinking" (Oh, 2005, p. 538) type of exchange or for an interrogation. In order for students to learn, the environment must be safe and allow them to question or say, "I don't know."

Often, when this type of questioning has identified the student's ZPD, either carefully worded questions to help the student build knowledge or direct instruction are warranted. Here, faculty should use their best judgment as to what the student needs in order to move on. A careful appraisal of the student's level of frustration, based on how his or her response post is worded, will shed light on the situation and best guide your strategy for responding.

Anderson and Piro (2014) suggested using Elder and Paul's Universal Intellectual Standards as a framework for building Socratic-style questions. These intellectual standards are clarity, accuracy, precision, relevance, depth, breadth, logic, and fairness (Elder & Paul, 1996). Questions associated with each standard to guide questioning in a purposeful manner can be found on Elder and Paul's website.

Toledo (2015) suggested that the wording of questions used in the Socratic method was very important as words perceived as harsh may result in students feeling intimidated and thereby the dialogue is ended. Probing questions are just that and if not phrased from the stance of caring and empathy, an emotional response from the student may be forthcoming when your intention was for a higher cognitive one. Using techniques of interpersonal communication, such as avoiding *you messages* and using *I messages* instead, will create less defensiveness. Also, softening the question and indicating your curiosity about what the student is thinking will indicate that, perhaps, you do not have all the answers and can learn from the student.

Stepien (1999) developed a list of questions grouped by intended outcomes that are based on the work of Richard Paul (Paul & Elder, 1996). These question starters are not only helpful for faculty, but also for students who can benefit from this approach, especially when questioning classmates to probe for deeper understanding. Toledo (2006) found that in sharing these questions with students as well as modeling the questions herself, she noted an improvement in the level of questions students asked each other, as well as the quality of the discussion. The questions developed by Stepien can be found on his website, the link to which is included in the reference to his work.

As mentioned earlier, the Socratic method is not a game of *guess what I am thinking.* It is also not asking random questions without purpose, a means to evaluate a student's performance, or a misguided opportunity to say "gotcha." The purpose of this method is to encourage critical thinking, identify the students' learning needs, and scaffold their learning (Oh, 2005). Scaffolding is another means of facilitation that is discussed later in this chapter.

Whiteley (2006) suggested combining the Socratic method with the cognitive domain of Bloom's taxonomy as a foundation for developing probing questions in response to students' posts. This seems like a valuable framework to help faculty determine at what level the student's understanding lies and at what level to begin questioning. Obviously, it is pointless to expect the students to analyze (analysis level of Bloom's cognitive domain) something if they do not understand (comprehension level) in the first place. This method involves naming the cognitive level that the student's post reflects and then posing higher level questions to advance the student's thinking toward a deeper level. My experience using this type of question during problem-based learning cases is that students quickly begin to mirror my behavior and ask more purposeful questions of each other.

Metacognitive Questioning

Metacognitive questioning is a method similar to the Socratic method in that probing questions are asked to promote deeper learning. The goal of metacognitive questioning is for faculty to model the type of questions they would ask themselves when thinking about an issue or solving a problem. Faculty then post this type of question in discussions when responding to students' questions so that soon students will ask themselves and others the same type of questions to guide their studying and learning.

Mevarech and Kramarski (2003) provided a framework for developing metacognitive questions in the IMPROVE method. This method was originally designed for teaching mathematics to junior high students; however, it is useful for our purposes. IMPROVE stands for a series of teaching steps: (a) introducing new concepts, (b) metacognitive questioning, (c) practicing, (d) reviewing, (e) obtaining mastery on lower and higher cognitive processes, (f) verification, and (g) enrichment (p. 451).

During the metacognitive questioning phase (the second step), students are taught to employ four kinds of metacognitive questions:

- *Comprehension questions* (e.g., What is the problem all about?)
- *Connection questions* (e.g., How is the given problem different from/similar to problems that have already been solved?)
- *Strategy questions* (e.g., What strategies are appropriate for solving the given problem and why?)
- *Reflection questions* (e.g., Does it make sense? Why am I stuck?) (p. 451).

Some of the wording of these questions is obviously related to the process of reviewing mathematical problems, but similar focused questions can be asked by faculty in a step-wise fashion to help students think through the problem.

Questions That Challenge

Using the facilitative technique of challenging students requires that students consider the discussions a place that is safe for them to speak their minds. Ng, Cheung, and Hew (2012) define challenging other students' contributions as "giving alternative suggestions/interpretations, pointing out gaps or discrepancies, or raising concerns about the points contributed by the participants" (p. 289). Challenging others' assumptions and arguments is necessary for productive discourse (Mezirow, 1997), but it must be done with respect and empathy. Mayer (1989, as cited in Toledo, 2015) recommends posing and wording questions based on the goal of developing trust. Asking a prior question of trust (PQT), as he termed it, involves considering "Is what I am doing, thinking, or saying, building trust or undermining trust?" (p. 276). I do think that asking oneself this question will ensure that you appropriately frame your response when challenging another's thoughts.

Stavredes (2011) reframed this type of question, calling it "taking another perspective" instead of challenging. Taking another perspective or playing devil's advocate gives students the opportunity to reflect on their perspective in light of another's and refine their position. When using this technique, I recommend starting the post with "I'm just playing devil's advocate here." Voicing appreciation for the student's perspective or acknowledging how it stimulated deeper thinking for you are other less confrontational ways to introduce your potentially conflicting opinion.

When topics are known to be controversial, Thomashow (1989, as cited in Thomas, 2005) established a series of questions to guide facilitation as well as students' approach to the topic—in essence to avoid "one-sided arguments" and/or "ill-informed opinions" (p. 112).

1. What is the controversy about?
2. What are the arguments?
3. What are the assumptions? Not all positions are valid if their arguments are based on prejudice or other flawed assumptions.
4. How are the arguments manipulated? Who is involved and what are their interests in the issue (p. 113)?

To the third point that Thomashow made, I would add the level of evidence included in the argument, an issue relevant to controversial issues in nursing practice.

Revoicing

According to O'Connor and Michaels (1993), revoicing is a facilitative technique used to restate, reframe, and recontextualize a conversation to focus on content and individual student's contributions. When two or more students are not in agreement, one option is to comment to one student that he or she is not in agreement with so and so and make an inference about the nature or degree of the disagreement. If faculty start the comment with "So . . .," the expectation is a response from all involved students giving them the opportunity to agree or disagree with what you have said and defend their individual positions. What this technique of "created opposition" does is place the involved students in an intellectual relationship for the time being and underscore the importance of the content of their posts. Other students reading this exchange will hopefully reflect on the various views as well and may, in fact, comment.

Another revoicing method is to restate what was said in language more appropriate to the discipline when the student has used more colloquial terms. This may involve using a larger umbrella term for what was said and reframing it to some degree, purposefully recontextualizing the comment. This approach again gives the student the opportunity to perhaps see the larger picture and affirm or deny your interpretation. In other words, "In this move, the teacher can take a student contribution and recast it within a wider frame or can slightly alter it to accent a different aspect of the lesson topic than the one intended by the student" (O'Conner & Michaels, 1993, p. 328). This is a useful technique to underscore a student's contribution who seems reluctant, shy, or is marginalized in some way.

Requesting Elaboration

Requesting elaboration is a frequent facilitative technique that involves asking the student to consider what he or she had posted at a deeper level. Questions to ask include "Can you say more about . . .?" or "Can you elaborate on your comment regarding . . .?" and then quote the comment. In a study by Ioannou, Demetrio, and Mama (2014), weakness of students' *initial* posts was often found to be a factor in knowledge construction as the discussion continued, especially when a student leader did not naturally emerge in the discussion to monitor and move the discussion forward. Even though the instructor facilitated the discussion using what appears to be elaboration in this study, two of the groups were less successful in constructing knowledge. Perhaps the take-away from this study, and mentioned by the authors as well, is that attention to elaboration-probing facilitation and monitoring responses from students is essential in the early stages of a discussion in order for it to be productive. Here I would reiterate that faculty involvement in a discussion should wait until all students post initially. If students do not respond to requests for more information, I would recommend a private e-mail be sent to determine potential issues. Perhaps, it is the case that the student's ZPD has been entered and he or she needs customized and personalized assistance in understanding the content, the discussion process, or the goal of the discussion.

Scaffolding

Education uses many metaphors based in the construction industry. We talk about construction of knowledge, building cognitive structures or mental models, writing a test blueprint, and scaffolding learning. From a construction perspective, a scaffold is a temporary structure, typically consisting of metal poles and wooden planks, that is built against the wall of a building so that workers can reach higher areas needing painting, for example, that they could not reach without the assistance a scaffold provides. As they complete the work higher up, the scaffold is gradually taken apart and lowered, and eventually eliminated altogether. Educational scaffolding works in much the same way. According to Wood, Bruner, and Ross (1976, as cited in Tudge & Scrimsher, 2003), who first used the term in an educational context involving younger children, scaffolding is a term that "consists essentially of the adult 'controlling' those elements of the task that are initially beyond the learner's capacity, thus permitting him to concentrate upon and complete only those elements that are within his range of competence" (p. 219).

As an example, let us look at how this might materialize in a discussion. Suppose you have noticed Mary's post is filled with direct quotes from the readings. That is what she can do on her own without guidance. This is her current ability with relation to this particular content or question posed. You post that while the information she has provided is interesting and relevant, you would like to read her own thoughts about the content as it relates or is applied to the DQ. Her reply post is apologetic and includes paraphrasing from the readings that indicate to you that she does not understand what she has read and/or cannot apply it. Taking the public conversation to a private space (e-mail or phone), you suggest that together you step back to review. Using questions from the metacognitive steps in the IMPROVE method (Mevarech & Kramarski, 2003) discussed in the Metacognitive Questioning section, you ask her to explain in her own words what the DQ is asking, a *comprehension level* question. Once you have helped her understand the question or realize she already does, you can move on to other question types from the metacognitive questioning phase.

The next question, a *connection* question, might ask her about how the readings relate to the DQ in her mind. Next would be a *strategy* question such as what content, concepts, and/or principles from the readings can be applied to the DQ. And, finally, a *reflection* question may be in order that asks the student to think about the proposed solution to the question or problem to determine if the fit is good.

Another related approach would be to use Bloom's taxonomy as the basis for asking questions to determine where the student's understanding ends. Begin with a *knowledge* question such as asking the student to define the terms in the DQ. Then, ask her to restate the question in her own words so you know that she understands it (comprehension). Next ask her to talk about what she learned from each of the readings, to determine if she understood what she read. If the DQ is written at the application level, ask how what she read might be applied to the DQ. If the question is written at a higher level of Bloom, use the verbs associated with those levels to help you formulate questions to stimulate the student's thinking.

So, how do you grade Mary's posts? Grading work that has been heavily scaffolded can prove challenging, but if the grading rubric assigns points to the initial post separately from responses to classmates, your task is made easier. Do you grade the first two poorly formulated posts? Let us suppose Mary is a dedicated student who, in previous discussions, has demonstrated that she wants to learn, and the scaffolding techniques you employed helped her find the right path. She has reposted her initial thoughts and it is now evident that she grasps the content and has gained understanding. Her learning is obvious. My perspective is that if the student's revised post demonstrates a better understanding of the material, I will grade that post. My approach is to grade the final product of learning and not deduct points because of the less than direct process it took to get there. However, it is important that you explain your rationales to Mary so it is not misinterpreted as giving points for effort, which is not a part of academic achievement, discussed in Chapter 9. You will, however, want to praise her for her hard work and stick-to-it attitude and willingness to wrestle with the content in order to understand. It is hoped that this will give her confidence and the issue will not repeat itself.

Scaffolding is a valuable facilitative tool to employ when students struggle to understand and apply what they have read to the DQ. As I mentioned earlier, recognizing the need for scaffolding is the first step. Posts that are difficult to understand (the blah-blah-blah post), less than substantive, full of quotes, or completely paraphrased without application to the question indicate that the student is struggling and faculty intervention by means of scaffolding is indicated.

Summarizing the Discussion

I often read about the recommendation for faculty to post some type of a wrap-up to each discussion in the form of a summary (Boettcher & Conrad, 2010). Another approach is to assign a different student in each group to summarize the discourse for their respective discussion groups. I see pros and cons of both recommendations.

Boettcher and Conrad (2010) offered several options when formally ending a discussion—what they considered "putting it to bed" (p. 150) and indicating the discussion is over. When posting a summary or closure post, be sure to label it "Wrap Up" or "Summary of Key Concepts" to alert students that you have reviewed their posts, are summarizing them, and will be offering your opinion. Alternatively, you can create a podcast and post it below the discussion board link within the week of the discussion. If either of these strategies is used, I recommend posting an announcement to let students know the summary has been posted, the form it is in (discussion post or podcast), and its location in the learning management system (LMS).

The downside of posting a summary is that it must be done quickly after the discussion has ended. Taking notes as you review students' posts throughout the discussion to include in the summary will make this task less of an effort. Quoting individual student's contributions to the discussion is a means of acknowledgment, especially when you preface the quote with something like "Jane mentioned in her initial post. . . ."

Asking each student to write a brief, two-to five-sentence summary of the discussion as a post, listing the take-away points he or she felt contributed most to learning, is another option and a pedagogically sound means of encouraging metacognitive strategies and reflection—a type of spaced study (see Chapter 1). Limiting the length of the posting is important as it forces students to reflect specifically on what they learned instead of summarizing, or even worse, reiterating the entire discussion.

Another recommendation by Boettcher and Conrad (2010) is to have one student summarize the discussion. Although this activity is pedagogically sound, logistically it is difficult. The student assigned to summarize must wait until the discussion end date and time have passed to review the posts and prepare a summary. Unless he or she has been taking notes throughout the discussion, this places a time-intensive burden on the student who may take several days to work on the summary post. If this summary is not posted in a timely fashion, other students in the group may have moved on to the next weeks' reading and do not return to the discussion board to review the summary. So, the summarizing student's effort may not be worth the time, given that few students may benefit from it. If you plan to have one student from each discussion group provide a summary, end the discussion on a Friday, for example, and have the summary post be due Sunday at midnight. I recommend that you review the course analytic logs typically available in most LMSs to track the number of students who returned to the discussion to read the summary post, whether it was your post or those of other students. Be objective in evaluating this practice and consider another approach if students are not reading the summaries.

CULTURAL CONSIDERATIONS

When teaching an online course in nursing, you will most likely have a mix of students from a variety of cultural backgrounds. Unfortunately, cultural identities are difficult to determine in the online environment as visual and aural clues are absent, potentially placing the instructor at a disadvantage. Including a cultural perspective in a discussion if appropriate to the topic may be an option to learn more about your students (Milheim, 2014). The insight from Garcia and Pearson (1991, as cited in Rovai, 2007) hit a cord with me. They said, "when teachers and majority culture students do not consider how students' cultural backgrounds affect their ways of communicating and working on a task, they tend to form false impressions about student abilities" (pp. 78–79). However, the flip side of this coin is that students who feel marginalized by their culture or race may feel liberated by this "racial cloaking," a term used by one of the faculty interviewed in Milheim's (2014, p. 5) study, knowing that assumptions cannot be made based on these variables. Sometimes students' names can indicate their cultural background, but that is far from a fool-proof method. I have found that students' grammatical errors, particularly subject-and-verb tense mismatches and syntax errors, are a tip-off that English is not their native language. These students often have difficulty understanding American jargon and colloquialisms, placing them at a disadvantage.

Ng et al. (2012) studied cultural influences among Asian Pacific graduate students during peer-facilitated critiques on their individual projects. The authors provided perspectives on how this cultural group might respond and communicate differently in discussions. This is relevant not only for faculty, but also for students, as they often take on the role of facilitator even if not assigned by faculty. The results indicated that:

- Showing appreciation for a student's feedback indicated that the facilitator was willing to hear opposing views, especially when the facilitator indicated he or she would reflect on the feedback.
- Open-ended questions gave them the freedom to provide personal opinions without the concern about being right or wrong.
- Challenging their perspective helped students construct new knowledge as long as the facilitator showed respect. However, Lim, Cheung, and Hew (2011) found that a post meant to challenge a student was misinterpreted and caused a student to withdraw from the discussion all together.
- Citing references decreased participation because it was viewed as a means to prove their perspectives were the right ones as they had a published author to agree with them. This could halt a discussion.

- Students felt that the instructor is the expert and should be respected and complied with.
- Challenging and criticizing others was considered culturally inappropriate. The students in this study avoided disagreement, especially with other students they did not know.
- Some withheld feedback because they did not want to offend a classmate.

THE TAKE-AWAY

Facilitation strategies are many, and applying them is an art, but is something that can be learned with time and practice. Key to choosing a useful facilitation strategy is assessing what is occurring in the discussion. It is particularly important to identify struggling students and intervene in such a way that they can overcome their learning issue and move forward to meet the outcomes of the discussion. Although research has not indicated what the ideal frequency of faculty involvement in a discussion is, current recommendations are to let your presence be known daily by posting briefly in each discussion group, posting an announcement, or replying to a student in Cybercafé, the place where students post general questions of interest. Tracking student progress in the discussions as well as your responses to students will save time and ensure that your presence indicates equal recognition and mutual awareness of all students.

REFERENCES

An, H., Shin, S., & Lim, K. (2009). The effects of different instructor facilitation approaches on students' interactions during asynchronous online discussions. *Computers & Education, 53*(3), 749–760.

Anderson, G., & Piro, J. (2014). Conversations in Socrates Café: Scaffolding critical thinking via Socratic questioning and dialogues. *New Horizons for Learning, 11*(1), 1–9. Retrieved from https://jhepp.library.jhu.edu/ojs/index.php/newhorizons/article/view/353

Boettcher, J. V. (2009). Have we arrived? *Campus Technology, 22*(8), 20–22.

Boettcher, J. V., & Conrad, R.-M. (2010). *The online teaching survival guide: Simple and practical pedagogical tips.* San Francisco, CA: Jossey-Bass.

Brown, P. C., Roediger, H. L., III, & McDaniel, M. A. (2014). *Make it stick: The science of successful learning.* Cambridge, MA: Belknap Press.

Burge, E. (2008, November). *Online issues carrying ethical implications.* Closing session, 14th Sloan-C International Conference on Online Learning, Orlando, FL.

Elder, L., & Paul, R. (1996). Universal intellectual standards. Retrieved from http://www.criticalthinking.org/pages/universal-intellectual-standards/527

Garrison, D. R., Anderson, T., & Archer, W. (1999). Critical inquiry in a text-based environment: Computer conferencing in higher education. *Internet and Higher Education, 2*(2–3), 87–105.

Garrison, D. R., & Arbaugh, J. B. (2007). Researching the community of inquiry framework: Review, issues, and future directions. *Internet and Higher Education, 10*(3), 157–172.

Hmelo-Silver, C. E., & Barrows, H. (2006). Goals and strategies of a problem-based learning facilitator. *Interdisciplinary Journal of Problem-Based Learning, 1*(1), 21–39. Retrieved from doi:10.7771/1541-5015.1004

Ioannou, A., Demetrio, S., & Mama, M. (2014). Exploring factors influencing collaborative knowledge construction in online discussions: Student facilitation and quality of initial postings. *American Journal of Distance Education, 28*, 183–195.

Lim, S. C. R., Cheung, W. S., & Hew, K. F. (2011). Critical thinking in asynchronous online discussion: An investigation of student facilitation techniques. *New Horizons in Education, 59*(1), 52–65.

Mevarech, Z. R., & Kramarski, B. (2003). The effects of metacognitive training versus worked-out examples on students' mathematical reasoning. *British Journal of Educational Psychology, 73*, 449–471.

Mezirow, J. (1997). Transformative learning: Theory to practice. *New Directions for Adults and Continuing Education, 74*, 5–12.

Milheim, K. L. (2014). Facilitation across cultures in the online classroom. *International Journal of Learning, Teaching and Educational Research, 5*(1), 1–11.

Moore, M. G. (1989). Three types of interaction [Editorial]. *American Journal of Distance Education, 3*(2), 1–7. doi:10.1080/08923648909526659

Ng, C. S., Cheung, W. S., & Hew, K. F. (2012). Interaction in asynchronous discussion forums: Peer facilitation techniques. *Journal of Computer Assisted Learning, 28*(3), 280–294.

O'Connor, M. C., & Michaels, S. (1993). Aligning academic task and participation status through revoicing: Analysis of a classroom discourse strategy. *Anthropology and Education Quarterly, 24*, 318–318.

Offir, B., Lev, Y., & Bezalel, R. (2008). Surface and deep learning processes in distance education: Synchronous versus asynchronous systems. *Computers & Education, 51*, 1172–1183.

Oh, D. C. (2005). The Socratic method in medicine: The labor of delivering medical truths. *Family Medicine, 37*(8), 537–539.

Reigeluth, C. M. (1999). What is instructional-design theory and how is it changing? In C. M. Reigeluth (Ed.), *Instructional-design theories and models* (Vol. II, pp. 5–30). Mahwah, NJ: Lawrence Erlbaum.

Rovai, A. P. (2007). Facilitating online discussions effectively. *Internet and Higher Education, 10*, 77–88.

Stavredes, T. (2011). *Effective online teaching: Foundations and strategies for student success.* San Francisco, CA: Jossey-Bass.

Stepien, B. (1999). Tutorial on problem-based learning: Taxonomy of Socratic questioning. Retrieved from http://ed.fnal.gov/trc_new/tutorial/taxonomy.html

Thomas, G. (2005). Facilitation in education for the environment. *Australian Journal of Environmental Education, 21,* 107–116.

Toledo, C. A. (2006). Does your dog bite? Creating good questions for online discussions. *International Journal of Teaching and Learning in Higher Education, 18*(2), 150–154.

Toledo, C. A. (2015). Dog bite reflections: Socratic questioning revisited. *International Journal of Teaching and Learning in Higher Education, 27*(2), 275–279.

Tudge, J., & Scrimsher, S. (2003). Lev S. Vygotsky on education: A cultural-historical, interpersonal, and individual approach to development. In B. J. Zimmerman & D. H. Schunk (Eds.), *Educational psychology: A century of contributions* (pp. 207–228). New York, NY: Routledge.

Whiteley, T. R. (2006). Using the Socratic method and Bloom's taxonomy of the cognitive domain to enhance online discussion, critical thinking, and student learning. *Developments in Business Simulation and Experiential Learning, 33,* 65–70.

12

Online Interface Design
and Course Management

You have made the major decisions on course design, including outcomes, assessments, and teaching strategies, using the Backward Design process (Wiggins & McTighe, 2005), and your syllabus has been completed. The one fairly large task remaining is the creation of the online course in the learning management system (LMS). This task requires a certain comfort with technology, but more important, consideration of interface design, or the computer–user interface with the goal of making the interface as user-friendly or intuitive as possible. Success in this endeavor depends on understanding the relationship of the syllabus and organization of the LMS. The focus of this chapter is to expand on the relationship of the syllabus to the LMS in order to create consistent navigation week after week that also maximizes the efficiencies available in most LMSs through understanding basic interface design principles.

THE LMS

All kinds of LMSs are currently available for use in higher education, with the names Blackboard and Moodle most recognizable. Technology is ever changing, and the new term you may have heard to replace LMS is the next-generation digital learning environments (NGDLE). The goals of moving to this environment are not only to digitalize the experience, but also to place learning at the center, which means customizing the experience for each learner depending on his or her learning needs (Brown, Dehoney, & Millichap, 2015).

For now, we will focus on LMSs that have similar functionality with the goal of creating an environment that is navigable and does not stand in the way of student learning. Because your syllabus must be reflected in how the LMS is set up or its look and feel, we will focus on that aspect first.

Keep in mind that two views of the LMS exist and are quite different—the student view and faculty view. Most LMSs allow you to switch to the student view to ensure that changes you have made are not only visible to students, but also look the way you had intended. It is good practice to check the course from the student view before the course starts.

ORGANIZING AN ONLINE COURSE

By Weeks or Modules?

The organization of the syllabus must parallel how the course is set up in the LMS, which was introduced in Chapter 3 in the section labeled Organization of an Online Syllabus. However, it is worth reiterating as doing so ensures that navigation will not get in the way of student's learning. Ideally, all courses in an academic program should follow the same schedule in that Week 1 starts on the first day of class and ends on the same day for all courses. Week 2 includes the same dates, and so on. This provides a stabilizing consistency for students that they seem to appreciate.

The LMSs that I am familiar with are organized in weekly segments that are automatically populated with the weekly dates for the entire course after you enter the start and end dates. They do not accommodate 2-week blocks. This can be problematic if you plan discussions that last 10 to 14 days. Consequently, using the concepts of modules or units that are guided by the content is the best approach, but the weeks should be listed in the syllabus. For the remainder of this chapter, I have used the term *module* to refer to 2 weeks of related content. For example, Module 1 may last for 2 weeks—Week 1 and Week 2. Organizing the syllabus by Module 1, Module 2, and so on will cause problems because it is not possible for the LMS to reflect that. Refer to Exhibit 3.2 (Chapter 3), under the section Organization of an Online Syllabus, which reflects the preferred organization of the course schedule so it is consistent with the setup of the LMS.

INTERFACE DESIGN

Interface design is also referred to as the computer–user interface. The LMS design should be intuitive and easily navigated so that students can focus on learning and not spend an undue amount of time locating information. User interface design "is the design of user interfaces for machines and software, such as computers, home appliances, mobile devices, and other

---

BOX 12.1
THREE GOLDEN RULES OF INTERFACE DESIGN

1. Place the user in control
2. Reduce cognitive load
3. Create a consistent interface

---

electronic devices, with the focus on maximizing usability and the user experience" (User Interface Design, 2016, para. 1). What we are concerned about is the functionality of the LMS software and what we can do with some predetermined choices to create an interface that is transparent.

Bahrami and Bahrami (2012) listed three golden rules of user interface design that appear in Box 12.1.

User Control

In order for the user, the learner in this case, to be in control, the navigation in the LMS should be consistent throughout the course. Using the same descriptive headings for each module creates consistency. These headings might include Introduction, Readings (required and recommended), Lectures, Discussions, and Assessments.

Introduction to the Module

For each module covering a 2-week time span, faculty should introduce the topic or theme in a podcast. Instead of using the title of Introduction, creative titles could be used for this introduction, such as Week at a Glance, The Week in Review, or Heads Up. When choosing a heading for the introduction, be consistent with your style of teaching and use the same titles for each module.

In Chapter 6, the topic of writing subobjectives was discussed, and I mentioned that this was not good practice in the new paradigm of nursing education. In the introductory podcast, I recommend including the following:

- The general learning outcomes for the module
- What prior knowledge students may have that is related
- How the learning outcomes will be achieved with the scheduled learning activities

- Any assignments that are due, with the location of the rubric to assess them
- Where the link to upload any assignments can be found
- Explanation of how the content they will be learning relates to their future role, providing examples if possible

This should provide a general overview of the module and allay any anxieties or answer any questions students may have. The link to the podcast should be included under the Introduction heading, or whatever you have decided to call that area.

Readings and Lectures

The syllabus includes reading assignments from the course text. If that is the only reading you will assign students, include the name of the text or the authors and the pages to be read for each module under the Readings heading. Some LMSs allow you to add text to the actual course homepage, but keep it to a minimum. If you have other readings, such as journal articles, copyright laws may prohibit you from uploading the article into your course. This varies by publisher, but instead of taking time to determine the rights for every article you want students to read, the best practice may be to add a direct link to the article in the school's library under the Readings heading. Consult your library for instructions on how to add a link for this purpose. Also, remember to indicate whether these readings are required or recommended using subheadings as part of the organizational framework of each module so students can plan their time.

Websites can be linked directly, but be sure to provide direction as to what you want students to do or read while they are there. It is too easy for students to get lost in cyberspace if specific directions are not provided. Using the back arrow on a browser will sometimes kick a student out of the LMS, requiring him or her to re-sign in, so do have the website as well as linked articles from the library open in a new window.

In a constructivist, learner-centered teaching paradigm, the lecture as the primary means of teaching has fallen out of favor, especially when teaching online. In addition, the millennial generation prefers a variety of teaching strategies (Price, 2009), and, although they prefer structure in educational activities (Wilson & Gerber, 2008), they prefer individual instruction or technology-based teaching strategies over the lecture (Mohr, Moreno-Walton, Mills, Brunett, & Promes, 2011). However, mini-lectures do have a place in online education. Mini-lectures should be reserved for complex topics that require more explanation than is provided in available published works, or to synthesize concepts and make connections that students may miss unless specifically pointed out. Creating and uploading long lectures that reiterate the text or other readings are not appropriate for the online environment, and, frankly, are a waste of your time. However, brief podcasts or YouTube videos are easy to create and provide a welcome reprieve from the text-based nature of online learning.

Links to Discussions

The learning space in most online courses is in the discussions. Links to the discussion forums can be set up from one main link under the discussion heading in each module. One sublink for each discussion group is then created. So, the main discussion link for each module would be Discussion 1, for example, indicating the first discussion in the course. Clicking on that link will allow you to set up a separate link for each group of students in the course. The advantage of this approach is to avoid multiple links to each discussion group appearing on the main page of the LMS, which takes up space and expands each week, requiring endless scrolling as the course progresses.

These sublinks for each group should be labeled with the discussion number and the group number. As discussions will most likely be graded, indicating a point value as a grade is part of setting up the discussions. When this occurs, the grade book is automatically populated with the same name used to set up the link and the point value of the assignment. If the discussion is not labeled with the discussion number and group number, these entries will all look the same to students when viewing the grade book from their perspective. So, the first discussion for Group 1 would be— Discussion 1, Group 1—or abbreviated as D1-G1. Brief abbreviations like this work well as the space for text in the grade book is limited.

Recall from Chapter 6 that one decision you will need to make is whether every group will tackle the same discussion question or if you will create different questions for each group. This is an important decision because you will need to set the discussion links you have created to either open for everyone in the class or be restricted to group members only. The other related decision you will need to make is whether a student can see the other posts by his or her classmates in the same discussion group before posting initially. Obviously, faculty want students to do their own work by completing the readings, synthesizing the information, and creating a unique post. If students can read each other's posts prior to posting, the risk is that they will essentially copy others' thoughts to create their own post. This is compounded if all groups are open for general viewing and working on the same discussion question. My recommendation is that if all groups are discussing the same question, you will want to (a) restrict access to the groups and (b) not allow students to see initial posts of other students in their group until they have posted for the first time. Note that these are separate steps in the setup procedure for discussion boards. This functionality is available when you set up the links and can be revisited at a later date to make adjustments, if needed.

Assessments

Not every module will include an assessment. However, when an assignment, such as a written paper, illness script, or podcast, is due, students will need to know where to upload it. The link to upload documents should be located in the week of the module that includes the due date for the assignment. For example, if an assignment is due February 5, and that date coincides with Week 5, the link should be placed under the heading of Assessments in Week 5. I would upload the rubric to grade this assignment under the assessment heading as well, even if it is included in the syllabus. A week or so prior to any assignment being due, it is recommended that you post an announcement reminding students of the upcoming assignment, when it is due, and where to upload it. At that time you can remind them that the rubric is in the syllabus and posted below the assignment's upload link. Students appreciate when faculty post information "just in time" that anticipates questions they have. This approach will save you time in the long run.

Managing Cognitive Load

Recall from Chapter 1 that *cognitive load* is the demand placed on learners' cognitive processing during learning (Miller, 2014). Extrinsic cognitive load relates to the unnecessary demands encountered that are not part of what is to be learned and can be influenced positively or negatively by design strategies faculty use to teach. Miller summarized the process: "When less cognitive power is taken up by extraneous load, more is left over for intrinsic and germane load" (p. 83), or those processes necessary for learning.

Multiple design strategies can reduce extrinsic cognitive load for students such as:

- *LMS orientation*
  An orientation to the LMS prior to the start or during the first week of classes that provides opportunities to practice with the features, such as posting in a discussion, uploading an assignment, and taking a practice quiz. This type of practice will allay anxieties even for those students who are familiar with and use other technologies often.

- *Use consistent course processes*
  - Assignments are due on the same day of the week and time. For example, all assignments are due Sunday night at 11:55 p.m.
  - Discussions start and end on the same day and at the same time. For example, all discussions start on Monday at 8:00 a.m. and end a week from the following Friday at 11:55 p.m.
- *Instructions are clearly written*
  Instructions for assignments and discussions are clearly spelled out in the syllabus and *just in time* weekly (at least) announcements remind students of upcoming activities.
- *Content is organized*
  The LMS is organized so that all components students need to complete a task are in the same place. For discussion, for example, the discussion question, length, due dates, and response requirements are visible when the student clicks on the main discussion link and again when he or she clicks on the group link to post.
- *Discussion questions are ill structured*
  Discussion questions that are ill structured and have no one correct answer are used consistently to decrease cognitive load as compared to questions for which answers can be found in the readings. The latter results in students all posting the same answer and struggling to find other things to say to meet the posting requirements.
- *Use varied formats for learning materials*
  Learning materials are presented in multiple modalities, when possible, such as a written script of a podcast, especially for complex content (Young, Van Merriënboer, Durning, & Ten Cate, 2014). Online learning is predominately a text-based medium and limiting all educational material to reading alone can cause cognitive overload and impair learning.
- *Provide worked examples when possible* (Van Merriënboer & Sweller, 2010)
  A worked example could be a complete history and physical exam write-up, letter to a senator, a brief, or worked statistical problems.
- *Hide future content*
  Most LMSs will allow you to hide content that students do not need to focus on. For example, you may have the entire course ready with all content uploaded before the start of the semester. Allowing students to see the entire course can be overwhelming and increase their anxiety and perhaps extrinsic cognitive load. Hide modules that students are not currently working on and open one module at a time, a week before the start date.

These are just a few suggestions to decrease extrinsic cognitive load. Basically, you want processes and extraneous information out of the way of learning for the student.

Consistent Interface Design

Consistent interface design of the LMS that includes the same headings in all weeks or modules, the same fonts and colors for headings, and the same processes week after week for posting in discussions and uploading assignments will impact extrinsic cognitive load by decreasing energy students must expend to figure things out, such as where to find needed items. When links are in the same place week after week, navigation is consistent and intuitive and extrinsic cognitive load is decreased.

Even students from the Net Generation who have been around technology most of their lives may find an LMS unfamiliar and need support learning the technology. As mentioned earlier, an orientation to the LMS that allows students to experiment with the functionality of the LMS in a nonthreatening environment will save faculty time answering questions. Also, creating how-to instructions that are available for students who need help will also save time answering questions later.

EFFICIENCIES

Teaching an online course can take most of your workweek if you do not control time spent. I have identified a number of efficiencies that will allow you to work smarter and save time when teaching online.

Cybercafé

The first efficiency that will save you a significant amount of time is to set up a discussion board link for the purpose of student questions. It is not really a chat area, as students will use instant messaging or Twitter if they want to converse with one another. The purpose of this discussion board, that could be named Cybercafé or Water Cooler, is for students to ask and answer questions to avoid sending you an e-mail. Students often have the same questions, so instead of receiving multiple e-mails that you must respond to individually, all students in the course can see the questions and your answers in Cybercafé. And, the beauty of this type of forum is that students will often answer the question for you, in which case it is important that you jump in as well, indicating agreement with the responding student, and thanking him or her for helping his or her classmate. When explaining the purpose of the Cybercafé to students, I mention that questions or concerns of a personal nature should be sent to my e-mail and I will respond.

Even with a Cybercafé in the course, students will e-mail you with routine questions that should have been posted in Cybercafé. Instead of telling them that, I answer the student's question and ask them to post the question and my response in Cybercafé. This serves several purposes; (a) the question and answer are posted for all to see, thus avoiding additional e-mails with the same question; (b) the student e-mailing you now understands the routine and feels comfortable posting in Cybercafé; and (c) other students will most likely comply with your request to use Cybercafé now that they see what will happen if they do not use it. A consistent approach in supporting students in using Cybercafé is essential or they will revert to e-mailing you with every question.

Just-in-Time Instruction

The concept of just-in-time pedagogy is based on Toyota's production system, which eliminated waste by producing "the necessary products in the necessary quantities at the necessary time" (Monden, 2011, p. 35). In other words, the software that ran the operation included a feedback loop that responded to subtle changes in demand that impacted all facets of production (raw materials, quantity of actual product, and storage) across all involved companies.

The notion of just-in-time teaching was subsequently developed (Gavrin, 2006) for the classroom, in which a feedback loop was established. This involved developing preclass exercises that students completed. Faculty then reviewed the responses prior to class and adjusted time spent in class on certain topics based on students' learning needs. Essentially, each class session was customized to meet the identified learning needs. How that relates to efficiencies is that after teaching a course a few times (and often based on faculty intuition), patterns of student learning needs emerge and faculty can anticipate where students will struggle, what specific information will be needed, and when it will be needed (Nelson, 1999). In the online environment, often students' learning needs can be understood from the questions they post in Cybercafé, which provide the information for the feedback loop.

Another approach also results in efficiencies for faculty. Instead of waiting for students to post questions in Cybercafé, many of these questions can be anticipated. If faculty post an announcement at the beginning of each week that reviews the week's activities, such as discussions and any assignments due (reiterated from the syllabus), briefly discusses how the reading will help the students, addresses why this topic is important to their continued learning and future role, and provides any additional information learned from semesters past, many yet-formed questions will be addressed and student anxieties allayed. If this is done consistently, students really appreciate the overview and reminder.

Remember that an announcement is a one-way communication from you to students. They cannot reply to your posts. For that reason, at the end of any announcement addressing a forthcoming module, I will remind students to post any questions they may have about what I have said or about the upcoming module in Cybercafé.

Online Calendar

Many LMSs include a calendar feature that allows faculty to add due dates for assignments and discussion posts. This feature serves as a summary of due dates from the syllabus in an online monthly calendar format to which students can add additional due dates to their personal view. Some LMSs can actually combine calendars for all courses the student is taking for a global, yet potentially cognitive overloading, view. Students appreciate the online calendar to plan their time and stay on task. For faculty, however, populating the calendar is often an additional step in preparing the online course. In some LMSs, when the upload links for assignments are set up, both the calendar and the grade book are populated, which is a very time-efficient feature.

Wikis

Many LMSs have a built-in wiki software that is fairly versatile. A wiki is like having a Word document online that everyone can edit. If you plan to have students collaborate on a final project as a result of a discussion group, they can do so in a wiki. The benefit of using this type of software is that students can edit one document instead of having to e-mail documents back and forth. When that occurs, invariably there are several versions floating around, and unless they are carefully labeled, you can quickly lose sight of which is the most current. A second advantage to having students work on projects in a wiki is that you can monitor the activity. If students choose different-colored fonts, you can easily identify and tell each student's contribution.

Wikis can also be used for course discussions. The benefit of this over a threaded discussion in a forum is that students can actually write in the middle of another student's post to ask a question or comment further. The conversation need not be linear. The downside of using a wiki for a discussion is that no time stamp occurs when students post, so unless they add the date and time, you cannot determine if they posted on time.

When you have students critique a peer's work, doing so in the wiki saves time. You can see the student's comments and provide feedback on them as well as on the work itself. Students can then copy and paste the paper above the initial version, delete the comments, and edit it in the wiki. This means setting up a wiki for each student dyad, which can be time-consuming.

The downside of a wiki is that in some LMSs if one person is editing his or her group's wiki, no one else can have access to it until the initial user exited the application. This can cause frustration if students compose their work within the wiki instead of copying and pasting it from another document. That is not always possible, however.

Overall, wikis are fairly easy to use and perfect for collaborative group projects, but do take some getting used to. Students may not like having to change the font color or really understand that adding a post does not need to be done at the end of the conversation. Providing detailed instructions up front is the best approach.

Course Adjustments for the Next Term

When you anticipate teaching the same course again, it is worthwhile to set up a means of tracking any changes that should be made as you discover them to help you when planning to teach the course again. After my syllabus is completed, I copy it, and place it in a folder labeled for the next semester and year I will teach the course. I also change the year on the syllabus to reflect when the course will be taught again, change the font of the year to red, and leave myself a note that this is a working syllabus. I can make any changes to that syllabus or make notes on it as I teach the course to avoid having to remember them later.

I also create and save a Word document that I title "Changes for [semester and year]." Then, any changes that come to me as I am teaching the course can either be made in the syllabus itself or as a note on that sheet. For example, I may receive an e-mail notification that a new edition of the text I have been using will be published and available before I teach the course the next time. I will make a note of that. Discussion questions or assignments that were not particularly successful in meeting learning outcomes, additional information needed when a module is taught again, or journal articles recently published that pertain to the topics are all stored in that folder. Then, when the time comes to teach the course again, I have a start on improving the course.

THE TAKE-AWAY

The importance of matching navigation in the LMS with how information is labeled in the syllabus cannot be overemphasized. Taking time to ensure this occurs will save you countless hours fielding questions from students and making changes once the course is underway. Taking advantage of efficiencies, such as Cybercafé and the online calendar, will also save precious time.

REFERENCES

Bahrami, M., & Bahrami, M. (2012). A review of software architecture for collaborative software's. *Advanced Materials Research, 433,* 2372–2376.

Brown, M., Dehoney, J., & Millichap, N. (2015, July–August). What's next for the LMS? *Educause, 17*(4), 9–18. Retrieved from http://er.educause.edu/articles /2015/6/whats-next-for-the-lms

Gavrin, A. (2006). Just-in-time teaching. *Metropolitan Universities, 17*(4), 9–18.

Miller, M. D. (2014). *Minds online: Teaching effectively with technology.* Cambridge, MA: Harvard University Press.

Mohr, N. M., Moreno-Walton, L., Mills, A. M., Brunett, P. H., & Promes, S. B. (2011). Generational influences in academic emergency medicine: Teaching and learning, mentoring, and technology (Part I). *Academic Emergency Medicine, 18*(2), 190–199.

Monden, Y. (2011). *Toyota production system: An integrated approach to just-in-time* (4th ed.). Boca Raton, FL: CRC Press.

Nelson, L. M. (1999). Collaborative problem solving. In C. M. Reigeluth (Ed.), *Instructional-design theories and models: A new paradigm of instructional theory* (pp. 241–267). Mahwah, NJ: Lawrence Erlbaum.

Price, C. (2009). Why don't my students think I'm groovy?: The new "R"s for engaging Millennial learners. *Teaching Professor, 23.* Retrieved from http://www .drtomlifvendahl.com/Millennial%20Charracturistics.pdf

User Interface Design. (2016). In *Wikipedia: The free encyclopedia.* Retrieved from https://en.wikipedia.org/wiki/User_interface_design

Van Merriënboer, J. J., & Sweller, J. (2010). Cognitive load theory in health professional education: Design principles and strategies. *Medical Education, 44*(1), 85–93.

Wiggins, G., & McTighe, J. (2005). *Understanding by design* (2nd ed.). Alexandria, VA: Association for Supervision and Curriculum Development.

Wilson, M., & Gerber, L. E. (2008, Fall). How generational theory can improve teaching: Strategies for working with the "Millennials." *Currents in Teaching and Learning, 1*(1), 29–44.

Young, J. Q., Van Merriënboer, J., Durning, S., & Ten Cate, O. (2014). Cognitive load theory: Implications for medical education: AMEE guide no. 86. *Medical Teacher, 36*(5), 371–384.

13

Tips for Converting a Classroom-Based Course to the Online Environment

DEFINITION OF *ONLINE LEARNING*

The definition of *online learning* has evolved over the years, but one definition is still not universally accepted. From my perspective, online learning has several defining characteristics. First, *synchronous* activity either online or face to face does not occur regularly as part of the course itself. Students may be required to attend on-campus residencies or immersions, but the weekly coursework is done within the learning management system (LMS). Second, and related to the first, is that the learning occurs in *asynchronous* small group discussions where students can coconstruct knowledge in a community of inquiry. Third, learning asynchronously supports reflective thinking, allowing time not only for independent research and reading of materials, but also for students to apply, analyze, synthesize, and/or evaluate what they have read in order to formulate a post for the discussion. And, finally, online education is anytime, anywhere learning. Blended online courses include a combination of classroom and online activity.

Distance education, on the other hand, is teaching and learning from a distance that typically includes a synchronous classroom setting in which students must be in front of a computer at certain times during the week. The main learning space is the online classroom, where students can actually see and hear each other. Although this offers the benefit of saving money by not having to drive to school and park, it is otherwise the same as attending class. This option requires thinking on one's feet and little time for research and reflection unless the questions have been provided ahead of the meeting. In a study by Chiasson, Terras, and Smart (2015), faculty who taught online courses using synchronous activity did not find any major differences as compared to teaching face to face. Thus, the modifications required to convert a classroom course to distance education required few changes in instructional strategies. This chapter focuses on the changes required when converting a classroom-based course to the online environment, that include the preceding characteristics of online teaching.

COURSE CONVERSION

Converting a face-to-face course to online can be a time-consuming process and one that is not necessarily given release time for faculty to complete. Time for revision is typically worked into a busy schedule as part of the faculty role (Chiasson et al., 2015) during the semester before you are scheduled to teach.

Let us consider how teaching online is different from teaching in a classroom. First, although discussions are important in the classroom to support learning, they cannot be assessed—at least not in a meaningful way unless you are using the clicker system, which records individual student responses to questions posed by the teacher. Online discussions, on the other hand, are pivotal to both assessment and learning. Second, class time takes on a broader meaning in the online environment, as it is anywhere, anytime. Gone is the worry of taking up valuable class time with quizzes that often served as a means of assessment only. Online, they become a meaningful teaching strategy. Third, lengthy lectures that reiterate the readings do not have a place in a constructivist paradigm—quite frankly online or in the classroom—but that notion has been slow to gain speed. Other teaching methods are far superior. Fourth, the playing field is somewhat leveled online. Everyone must participate if discussions are a part of the course. This is beneficial on two fronts. First, as faculty you can readily see who understands and can apply the content and who is struggling. In addition, participation does not rely on one's verbal skills and the ability to think quickly. In online discussions, time for reading, assimilating the content, and reflecting exists.

Revisiting the Backward Design Process

Course revision is best accomplished by following the steps in the Backward Design process as originally developed by Wiggins and McTighe (2005), which I reconceptualized for teaching online. The two steps used to develop online courses are (a) identifying outcomes, and (b) determining students have met the learning outcomes (assessments) by authentic means that also double as methods of teaching.

Writing objectives is often the first step, but as they are already in place in the classroom-based version of the course, the same objectives must be used for the online course in order for the courses to be considered equivalent academically. So, your job is to interpret the existing objectives to determine appropriate assessment strategies and teaching methods for the online environment. Initially, your focus should be on assessing the learning outcomes reflected in the objectives.

Keep in mind that what are considered strictly assessments when teaching in a classroom, double as teaching methods online. Discussion boards and quizzes can serve as both. Because of this you may not need to devise additional assessment methods to assess the objectives, which decreases your workload. Avoid busywork for students by getting all the mileage you can from discussions, quizzes, drill-and-practice exercises, and additional methods that do support the construction of knowledge, long-term transfer, and learning (Roediger & Karpicke, 2006).

What About the Lecture?

Unlike teaching in a classroom, the lecture takes second stage to other methods of teaching and learning. Lectures cannot simply be uploaded to the LMS and be considered "teaching online." When reminiscing about a former professor's advice, Pelz (2004) mentioned that "a lecture is the best way to get information from the professor's notebook into the student's notebook without passing through either brain" (p. 33). The content from lectures already created for the classroom, however, can provide a basis for creating quiz questions and perhaps identifying complex content that students often struggle to understand. Mini-lectures in a podcast or YouTube video are useful for teaching complex content or when you want to be sure students make connections between concepts or content.

Students often welcome mini-lectures that explain challenging content via a different approach that is complementary to the assigned readings. Repeating what is in the text or outlining a chapter is not typically helpful or welcomed. Podcasts, voice-over PowerPoints, or YouTube videos are means of presenting these mini-lectures. Keep in mind that audio and video files are large and often exceed the limits of the uploading ability of most LMSs.

YouTube videos can easily be created using screen capture software such as iShowU, which can be purchased for a reasonable price as of this writing. However, searching the Internet for screen capture software compatible with the operating system on your computer that can be converted into a YouTube video is another means of learning what is available. Screen capture software allows you to record your lecture using the microphone built into your computer while viewing the PowerPoint lecture on your desktop that you developed. Be sure to run the PowerPoint in slideshow view mode so it takes up your entire desktop. With the software, a few clicks will convert what you have recorded into a YouTube video.

With a Google account, you can create your own library on YouTube and upload the videos you have created. This allows you to add a link to your course instead of uploading a large multi megabyte voice-over PowerPoint lecture that will not only take up space in the LMS, but also increase download time prior to viewing. In the settings menu for each video you upload to YouTube, you can set it for private or public viewing.

A podcast can also be created using the screen capture software, but keep in mind that whatever is on your desktop will be recorded. A way to get around this is to create a one-slide PowerPoint presentation that lists the name of the podcast, the author's name, and the date. Setting PowerPoint on slideshow view will cover up anything on your desktop while you record. Remember to close other applications, so a pop-up of an incoming e-mail does not interrupt your recording session. Adding the link of a YouTube video (or audio file) without actually embedding it in the LMS software allows flexibility in the file size you create. Students can then download the MP3 file you have created and listen to it on the go.

Podcasts can also be created using GarageBand on a Mac or QuickTime player on either a PC or Mac. Remember that Audacity (Audacity, n.d.) is a free, user-friendly download used to record MP3 files. Students seem to find listening to a mini-lecture instead of reading about it, a welcome relief from the text-based nature of online education.

If mini-lectures are part of your course, be sure to include quiz questions to see if students have learned the content. Creating these lectures is time consuming, so extrinsically motivating students to listen to them by quizzing them on the content or working it into a discussion is warranted.

Small Group Discussions

I do hope that after reading Chapters 6 and 7 you understand how important small group discussions are as a space in which students can co-construct knowledge. However, creating discussion questions or cases that are engaging is required. But once that is accomplished, I think you will be amazed at how students jump into the role and begin to think like a nurse practitioner (NP), researcher, administrator, or educator as they wrestle with the problem or dilemma you have created for them.

A great deal of bad press exists in academia about how time consuming teaching online can become. That has not been my experience when courses are designed with workload in mind, assessments and teaching methods are chosen for their dual role, and additional learning activities are created using software in the LMS that runs itself.

So, do consider discussions as the main learning space in your course regardless of the content you will be teaching. Take some time to consider *why* they are learning the content from your course and *how* will it be used in their future role. That is the place to start. Other suggestions presented in Chapters 6 and 7 will help you design authentic questions or cases.

Quizzes

Whenever possible take advantage of the testing effect (Chapter 1, The Testing Effect and Spaced Study section) by offering frequent online quizzes that include feedback for incorrect answers, allow multiple attempts to achieve mastery, and can deliver a variety of levels of questions. Assign a few points to these quizzes as extrinsic motivation so students will take them seriously. Lower level cognitive questions are useful in activating what the student already knows, but perhaps has not thought about for many years. Bringing forward that knowledge stored in mental models helps to strengthen the cues for retrieval as well as allows new, related content to be added to the schema, enriching it. In addition, cognitively staged questions (Chapter 8) will help you identify students' zone of proximal development so you can provide remediation if needed.

Because online testing cannot be monitored without a great deal of planning, I recommend that you avoid using tests as summative assessments. The safeguards that are present in the classroom, such as ensuring students do not consult their texts while taking the test, collaborate on answers, or simply look at their neighbor's answers, are not available for online testing. You can remind students that cheating is considered academic dishonesty, a violation of the honor code, and could result in them being expelled from school, but you really cannot know with certainty what went on while they were taking the test. Cognitive science research validating the value of the testing effect is very compelling, so using these quizzes for formative assessment has value.

Other Means of Teaching and Assessment

Additional assessments appropriate for online courses are listed in Chapter 3. However, I encourage faculty to be creative in assessing and teaching. Attributes of an assessment from a constructivist paradigm include authentic content set in an authentic context; multiple perspectives, that is, no one right answer; requiring at the minimum application-level thinking; and quizzes that provide the right answer for incorrect responses.

Trying a new assessment or teaching method is often not done because of the potential consequences of negative end-of-course survey responses from students. The key to avoiding this is in developing a collegial relationship with your students and communicating your rationales to them. Do follow-up and ask for feedback regarding the new teaching method or assessment before too much time has lapsed and certainly before the end-of-course surveys have been distributed. Do so with an anonymous online survey so students will be honest. The anonymity of the survey will also alleviate any concerns students may have regarding retaliation from you if their comments are negative.

Some Practical Advice

Pelz (2004), a very practical yet theory-driven professor, shared his three principles of online pedagogy, which I must admit I agree with. His first principle is "let the students do (most of) the work" (p. 33). Most faculty realize that even though we *teach* students, they must do the learning. We cannot make them learn. What we can do is have high expectations of students and communicate that. They will often rise to the occasion. Engaging discussion questions, case-based learning activities, and authentic assignments that place them in the role they are studying for put them in a position to use the type of reasoning required in that role. Somehow that is empowering to students. They will take the ball and run with it and all I need to do is watch, keep them on track, and pull them back when they stray.

Pelz's (2004) second principle is that "interactivity is the heart and soul of effective asynchronous learning" (p. 37). His advice is to create opportunity for meaningful interaction such as engaging discussions, collaborative group discussions, or authentic group projects. Provide specific details of the activity along with the expectations in a rubric. Demonstrate that you are available by responding quickly to students' questions in the Cybercafé.

Pelz's (2004) third principle is to "strive for presence" (p. 41). I like his choice of verb as it indicates that what we may consider presence may not meet the students' expectation of how often we should post. However, being aware of the community of inquiry model (Garrison, Anderson, & Archer, 1999) of social, cognitive, and teaching presence (Chapter 10), the strategies recommended that demonstrate each, and useful methods to support students in development of these presences will provide a framework for being present for your students.

Support When Troubles Arise

When converting a classroom-based course to the online environment, you will need various kinds of support (Chiasson et al., 2015; El-Naga & Abdulla,

2015). Knowing what kind of support you need and whom to turn to is half the battle. You may need to find colleagues who can assist you with designing the online course, implementing best practices in terms of pedagogy, and learning the technical aspects of the LMS. Most likely, you will not find one person who can help you with all these tasks.

If technology is the issue, the information technology (IT) department can help. It is to be hoped that they have provided how-to videos or step-by-step instructions to help you set up the LMS, upload files, and set up the grade book. If not, they should be available to help you with these tasks as well as troubleshoot throughout the semester, should problems arise. If the LMS is not meeting your needs, the IT administrator may be able to address the issue. Sometimes the desired functionality exists in the LMS, but the top level IT administrator has it turned off, thinking it is not useful. Remember that those who administer the LMS are most likely IT folks, not pedagogy experts. You will need to let them know what you need. To illustrate this point, Chiasson and colleagues (2015) interviewed 10 faculty members about their experiences transitioning their face-to-face course to the online environment. The authors noted, "what was interesting about the participants in this study was the need for continuous support, yet there was an underlying passivity for improving institutional support" (p. 237). I think this stems from two interrelated problems. First, faculty do not really know what kind of support they need, so they do not ask. I jokingly said to more than one faculty when I was in an instructional design position that they *could not tell me what they didn't know*. It's true! However, if you start asking questions, you will find the type of support you need. Second, faculty are reluctant to admit to not knowing what they think they should know. My experience taught me that when a faculty member was unable to figure something out in the LMS, instead of asking me a question so I could walk them through how to fix the problem, they would rather spend hours trying to figure it out themselves. Why do that when you can pick up the phone and talk to someone more knowledgeable in that particular area? Please use what resources you have available to you. I realize you are most likely an expert classroom teacher, but a novice teaching online. We all started out as novices; experts are rarely born.

If you are having difficulty with course design, an instructional designer (ID) is the expert in that area. They are the teaching methods experts. Working with you, the content expert, an ID can ask the appropriate questions and make suggestions on the best approach to teaching. I realize that not all institutions have these various types of support available. IDs are rare in colleges of nursing. However, the university or college may have an ID available.

THE TAKE-AWAY

Faculty often feel intimidated when designing their first online course and are hesitant to ask for help and uncertain whom to turn to. Online course design follows the same basic steps that are completed to create an outcome-based classroom course. However, understanding the differences between teaching online and in the classroom, especially the dual role of assessments and teaching methods, is paramount to managing workload for both you and your students.

REFERENCES

Audacity® [Computer software] SourceForge. Retrieved from http://www.audacityteam.org

Chiasson, K., Terras, K., & Smart, K. (2015). Faculty perceptions of moving a face-to-face course to online instruction. *Journal of College Teaching & Learning, 12*(4), 231–240.

El-Naga, N. A., & Abdulla, D. (2015). A roadmap to transform learning from face-to-face to online. *Journal of Education and Training, 2*(1), 168–183.

Pelz, B. (2004). (My) three principles of effective online pedagogy. *Journal of Asynchronous Learning Networks, 8*(3), 33–46.

Roediger, H. L., & Karpicke, J. D. (2006). The power of testing memory: Basic research and implications for educational practice. *Perspectives on Psychological Science, 1*(3), 181–210.

Wiggins, G., & McTighe, J. (2005). *Understanding by design* (2nd ed.). Alexandria, VA: Association for Supervision and Curriculum Development.

Appendix:
Curriculum Design
Templates

These templates can be downloaded from the Springer Publishing Company website at www.springerpub.com/kennedy.

TEMPLATE 4.6
Course-Alignment Template for Use When Writing Objectives

Outcomes	Objectives—*At the End of This Course, the Students Will Be Able to:*	Assessments	Teaching strategies

TEMPLATE 4.7
Course-Alignment Template for Use When Interpreting Objectives

Course description:
Objectives:

Objective Number	Assessments	Teaching Strategies

TEMPLATE 6.3
Course Content Map

Case Number	Foreground Content	Background Information			
	Chief complaint given to students:	Professional context:			
	Diagnosis for this case:				
	Diagnoses for other cases:				
	Potential diagnoses: (Peripheral domain content)	Comorbidities	Meds/Allergies	Social History	Family History
Case Number	Foreground Content	Background Information			
	Chief complaint given to students:	Professional context:			
	Diagnosis for this case:				
	Diagnoses for other cases:				
	Potential diagnoses: (Peripheral domain content)	Comorbidities	Meds/Allergies	Social History	Family History
Case Number	Foreground Content	Background Information			
	Chief complaint given to students:	Professional context:			
	Diagnosis for this case:				
	Diagnoses for other cases:				
	Potential diagnoses: (Peripheral domain content)	Comorbidities	Meds/Allergies	Social History	Family History

TEMPLATE 6.4
Cognitive Case Map

	Initial Content Provided	Connections
Case Number		
Chief complaint given to students:		
Professional context:		
Expected list of potential diagnoses:		
Content Provided as Case Unfolds		
History		
Exam		
Lab		
Assessment		
Plan		

TEMPLATE 6.5
Illness Script

Case:

Working Hypothesis	Predisposing Conditions	Pathophysiological Insult	Discriminating Features (Such as Expected Findings on the History and Exam)	Defining Feature or Qualifier

PhD Discussion Question Development Worksheet

Name of course:
Program of study:
Numbered objectives for course:

DQ	Problem or Issue	Foreground Content	Background Content	Professional Context	Objective Number Assessed
1					
2					
3					
4					
5					
6					
7					
8					

DQ, discussion question.

TEMPLATE 7.2
RN to Bachelor of Science in Nursing (BSN) Discussion Question
Development Worksheet

Name of course:
Program of study:
Numbered objectives for course:

Problem or issue:
Foreground content:
Background content:
Professional context:
Subcontext—
Discussions:

TEMPLATE 7.3
Nonclinical Course Discussion Question Development Worksheet

Name of course:
Program of study:
Numbered objectives for course:

DQ	Problem or Issue	Foreground Content	Background Content	Professional Context	Objective Number Assessed
1					
2					
3					
4					
5					

DQ, discussion question.

TEMPLATE 7.4

NP Discussion Question Development Worksheet

Name of course:
Program of study:
Numbered objectives for course:

DQ	Problem or Issue	Foreground Content	Background Content	Professional Context	Objective Number Assessed
1					
2					

DQ, discussion question.

Module 1	
DQ:	
Content	Connections

Module 2	
DQ:	
Content	Connections

Module 3	
DQ:	
Content	Connections

Module 4	
DQ:	
Content	Connections

Module 5	
DQ:	
Content	Connections

Module 6	
DQ:	
Content	Connections

Module 7	
DQ:	
Content	Connections

Module 8	
DQ:	
Content	Connections

DQ, discussion question.

TEMPLATE 8.1
Test Blueprint

Course:
Semester/Year:
Objectives:

	Cognitive Objectives					
	1	2	3	4	5	Total
Knowledge						
Comprehension						
Application						
Analysis						
Synthesis						
Evaluation						
Totals						

TEMPLATE 11.1
Discussion-Tracking Tool

Names of Students	Discussions									
	1		2		3		4		5	
	I	R	I	R	I	R	I	R	I	R

I, initial post; R, response post.

Index